Skull Base Surgery - Pearls and Nuances

Edited by Amit Agrawal

Published in London, United Kingdom

Skull Base Surgery - Pearls and Nuances
http://dx.doi.org/10.5772/intechopen.1000398
Edited by Amit Agrawal

Contributors
Abdul Hye Manik, Ahmed-Ul-Mursalin Chaudhury, Ali Awad, Amir Alim, Amit Agrawal, Deepak Krishna, Hasnain Faisal, Haytham Osman, Honida Ibrahim, Khalid Elzein, Manal M. Khan, Md Al Amin Salek, Nazik Abdullah, Nwoshin Jahan, Rahul Dubepuria, Rajib Sahriar, Rukun Uddin Chowdhury, Shamantha Afreen, Trung Kien Duong

First published in London, United Kingdom, 2024 by IntechOpen
IntechOpen is the global imprint of INTECHOPEN LIMITED, registered in England and Wales, registration number: 11086078, 167-169 Great Portland Street, London, W1W 5PF, United Kingdom

British Library Cataloguing-in-Publication Data
A catalogue record for this book is available from the British Library

Additional hard and PDF copies can be obtained from orders@intechopen.com

Skull Base Surgery - Pearls and Nuances
Edited by Amit Agrawal
p. cm.
Print ISBN 978-0-85466-359-0
Online ISBN 978-0-85466-358-3
eBook (PDF) ISBN 978-0-85466-360-6

For EU product safety concerns:
IN TECH d.o.o., Prolaz Marije Krucifikse Kozulić 3, 51000 Rijeka, Croatia, info@intechopen.com or visit our website at intechopen.com.

Meet the editor

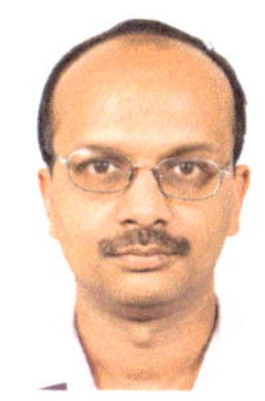

Dr. Amit Agrawal completed his neurosurgery training at the National Institute of Mental Health and Neurosciences, Bangalore, India, in 2003. He is a self-motivated, enthusiastic, and results-oriented professional with more than 20 years of rich experience in research and development and teaching and mentoring in neurosurgery. He is proficient in managing and leading teams for running successful process operations and has experience developing procedures and service standards of excellence. He has attended and participated in many international and national symposiums and conferences and delivered lectures on vivid topics. He has published more than 750 articles in national and international journals. His expertise is in identifying training needs, designing training modules, and executing the same while working with limited resources. He has excellent communication, presentation, and interpersonal skills with proven abilities in teaching and training for various academic and professional courses. Presently, Dr. Agrawal is working at the All-India Institute of Medical Sciences, Bhopal, Madhya Pradesh, India.

Contents

Preface

Over the years, with advancements in imaging and management techniques, the domain of skull base surgery has expanded enormously, dealing with pathologies extending their reach into neighboring territories such as the orbits, paranasal sinuses, craniocervical junction, and the head-neck region involving the bony skull, brain and its covering, cranial nerves, major cerebral vessels, venous sinuses, and the brainstem. The spectrum of techniques encompasses traditional open approaches with ever-growing precision of endoscopic methods, supplemented with a multidisciplinary team of specialists. This book selectively discusses the complex terrain of skull base surgery and elaborates on approaches to the anterior, middle, and posterior cranial fossa. The introductory chapter provides a comprehensive overview of penetrating skull base injuries, discussing their etiology, clinical presentation, diagnostic workup, and management strategies. Other chapters discuss transnasal endoscopic pituitary surgery, including its indications, techniques, and potential complications; the endoscopic endonasal approach for tuberculum-planum sphenoidale meningioma; reconstruction of scalp and forehead defects; and management of blunt cerebrovascular injury. This book contributes to existing knowledge for the management of complex pathologies involving the skull base and related structures.

Amit Agrawal
Department of Neurosurgery,
All India Institute of Medical Sciences,
Bhopal, India

Chapter 1

Introductory Chapter: Penetrating Skull Base Injuries

Amit Agrawal

1. Introduction

Penetrating skull base injuries (PSBI) can be caused by a range of mechanisms, and present a diagnostic and management challenge [1–5]. Usually, these injuries are caused by sharp objects, and these objects get entry into the skull via oro-cranial, transorbital intracranial, or transnasal routes [6–8]. While examining this group of patients, a high index of suspicion as if the entry wound is small, these lesions can be overlooked, hence, the overall incidence may get under-reported [4, 9]. A range of objects have been reported to cause PSBI raging from toilet brush handle, arrows, chopsticks, flatware, screwdrivers, keys, car antenna aerials, scissors, knives, pitch-forks, crochet hooks, knitting needles, breech pins, umbrella bibs, crowbars, and iron rods [4–7, 10–18]. There is an ongoing need to better understand PSBIs including associated complications, and to develop effective management protocols for these sub-groups of traumatic brain injuries [1, 19–24].

2. Epidemiology

In view of low incidence, the overall epidemiology is largely compiled from reported cases and experiences from different institutions [4, 25–29]. Common causes of PSBIs include accidents, suicide attempts, and assaults [30], accounting for approximately 0.4% of all cases of head injuries [31]. The risk of injuries is higher in children who may be left unattended due to various reasons or attended by younger siblings [32]. PSBIs can be caused by low-velocity projectiles, i.e. the impact velocity < 100 m/s [33]. In cases of PSBIs, the foreign bodies can penetrate the cranial cavity via the orbital roof route as the orbital plate of the frontal bone, through face and facial bones, through the nasal cavity, or may directly penetrate the skull bones if the force is strong enough [5, 16, 18, 21, 34–36].

3. Imaging

In addition to careful and systematic clinical examination, radiological imaging has improved our approach to detect PSBIs as it will show the presence and route of foreign bodies and, extent of injury to bones and brain parenchyma [21]. The modalities of imaging include CT scan (including 3-D reconstruction) with bone window, MRI, X-ray skull, and in ocular route of entry, the ultrasound imaging of the orbit and its contents [1, 37]. The presence of radiopaque foreign bodies including metallic

IntechOpen

foreign bodies can be well visualized on CT scan and radiographs, however, organic foreign bodies including peanut, wood, or bamboo pieces may be missed [4–6, 38–40]. Non-metallic foreign bodies can be better visualized on contrast-enhanced magnetic resonance imaging (MRI) [41, 42]. CT angiogram is to assess the cerebral vasculature as well as the magnitude of bone loss or damage during these injuries [1].

4. Management

A combination of careful history, clinical examination, radiological imaging, and high index of suspicion can help in planning the comprehensive management of patients with PSBIs [40]. Once the details of the trajectory of foreign body, presence of absence including the site of CSF leak and the details and associated intracranial hematomas or vascular injuries are obtained, a strategy to treat conservatively or surgical approaches can be planned [1, 28, 35, 43, 44]. The basic principles are early removal of foreign (to reduce the risk of infection), removal of foreign body, and meticulous repair of the defect particularly of the dura to stop or prevent CSF and reduce the risk of meningitis and other catastrophic complications [6, 8, 21, 28, 40, 45, 46]. This can be followed by broad-spectrum antibiotics based on the institute policy or available guidelines, which can be changed to appropriate antibiotics after the culture and sensitivity report is available [6, 40, 47–49].

5. Complications

PSBI can be associated with various complications including intracranial infections, cerebrospinal fluid leaks, intracranial hemorrhage, pneumocephalus, and cerebral edema [2–5]. Appropriate antibiotics can be selected aiming to manage the *Staphylococcus aureus* and Gram-negative organisms as these are the most common organisms, later can be changed to the antibiotics based on culture and sensitivity patterns [16, 30, 47, 50, 51]. It is of utmost importance to anticipate the potential risk of CSF leak and take adequate measures to repair the defects in bone and remove the foreign bodies [1, 6, 52–54]. The complications can be potentially prevented by appropriate and timely management interventions including careful and thorough irrigation of the wound to remove contaminated bone and tissue fragments and any foreign bodies [30, 35]. Post-operative imaging particularly a CT scan brain can be performed to ensure the removal of foreign bodies or any new or expanding parenchymal hematomas [55, 56].

6. Conclusions

In summary, regular follow-up with patients who have PSBIs can help recognize any infection complications or CSF leaks. If the patient has sustained subtle vascular injuries, a high index of suspicion and appropriate investigations like CT angiography can help to diagnose the formation of pseudoaneurysms or any delayed intracranial hemorrhages [30, 57–60]. Patients prone to post-traumatic acute stress or adaptive disorder can be subjected to a comprehensive psychiatric assessment and can be managed if there are signs of distress [30]. Although PSBIs due to low-energy penetrating injuries are not common, knowledge and understanding of the mechanism and management of these injuries are important to achieve favorable outcomes. The management of PSBIs requires recognition of subtle external injuries, understanding of clinical approach algorithms, available management options, and the spectrum of complications, as these will help to decide the optimal treatment approach for each individual patient.

Author details

Amit Agrawal
Department of Neurosurgery, All India Institute of Medical Sciences, Bhopal, Madhya Pradesh, India

*Address all correspondence to: dramitagrawal@gmail.com; dramitagrawal@hotmail.com

References

[1] Lan Z, Richard SA, Ma L, Yang C. Nonmissile anterior Skull-Base penetrating brain injury: Experience with 22 patients. Asian Journal of neurosurgery. 2018;**13**(3):742-748

[2] Chowdhury FH, Haque MR, Hossain Z, Chowdhury NK, Alam SM, Sarker MH. Nonmissile penetrating injury to the head: Experience with 17 cases. World Neurosurgery. 2016;**94**:529-543

[3] Li XS, Yan J, Liu C, Luo Y, Liao XS, Yu L, et al. Nonmissile penetrating head injuries: Surgical management and review of the literature. World Neurosurgery. 2017;**98**(873):e9-e25

[4] Sweeney JM, Lebovitz JJ, Eller JL, Coppens JR, Bucholz RD, Abdulrauf SI. Management of nonmissile penetrating brain injuries: A description of three cases and review of the literature. Skull Base Reports. 2011;**1**(1):39-46

[5] Turbin RE, Maxwell DN, Langer PD, Frohman LP, Hubbi B, Wolansky L, et al. Patterns of transorbital intracranial injury: A review and comparison of occult and non-occult cases. Survey of Ophthalmology. 2006;**51**(5):449-460

[6] Teng TS, Ishak NL, Subha ST, Bakar SA. Traumatic transnasal penetrating injury with cerebral spinal fluid leak. EXCLI Journal. 2019;**18**:223-228

[7] Agrawal A, Pratap A, Agrawal CS, Kumar A, Rupakheti S. Transorbital orbitocranial penetrating injury due to bicycle brake handle in a child. Pediatric Neurosurgery. 2007;**43**(6):498-500

[8] Arslan M, Eseoglu M, Gudu BO, Demir I. Transorbital orbitocranial penetrating injury caused by a metal bar. Journal of Neurosciences in Rural Practice. 2012;**3**(2):178-181

[9] Mason F. Case of a young man who had a pitchfork driven into his head four inches who speedily got well. Lancet. 1870;**1**:700-701

[10] Pilcher C. Penetrating wounds of the brain: An experimental study. Annals of Surgery. 1936;**103**(2):173-198

[11] Gennarelli TA, Champion HR, Sacco WJ, Copes WS, Alves WM. Mortality of patients with head injury and extracranial injury treated in trauma centers. The Journal of Trauma. 1989;**29**(9):1193-1201; discussion 201-2

[12] Hayashi Y, Fujisawa H, Tohma Y, Yamashita J, Inaba H. Penetrating head injury caused by bear claws: Case report. The Journal of Trauma. 2003;**55**(6):1178-1180

[13] Smrkolj V, Balazic J, Princic J. Intracranial injuries by a screwdriver. Forensic Science International. 1995;**76**(3):211-216

[14] Tutton MG, Chitnavis B, Stell IM. Screwdriver assaults and intracranial injuries. Journal of Accident & Emergency Medicine. 2000;**17**(3):225-226

[15] Ward JD, Chisholm AH, Prince VT, Gilman CB, Hawkins AM. Penetrating head injury. Critical Care Nursing Quarterly. 1994;**17**(1):79-89

[16] Bayston R, de Louvois J, Brown EM, Johnston RA, Lees P, Pople IK. Use of antibiotics in penetrating craniocerebral injuries. "Infection in Neurosurgery" Working Party of British Society for

Antimicrobial Chemotherapy. Lancet. 2000;**355**(9217):1813-1817

[17] Soose RJ, Simons JP, Mandell DL. Evaluation and management of pediatric oropharyngeal trauma. Archives of Otolaryngology – Head & Neck Surgery. 2006;**132**(4):446-451

[18] Sun G, Yagmurlu K, Belykh E, Lei T, Preul MC. Management strategy of a transorbital penetrating pontine injury by a wooden chopstick. World Neurosurgery. 2016;**95**(622):e7-e15

[19] Hebecker R, Sola S, Lenz JH, Just T, Piek J. An unusual case of a penetrating skull-base injury caused by a wild deer's antler. Central European Neurosurgery. 2009;**70**(1):48-51

[20] Onyekwe LO, Ohaegbulam SC. Penetrating orbito-cranial and ocular cow-horn injuries. Nigerian Journal of Clinical Practice. 2007;**10**(2):177-179

[21] Yuan YK, Sun T, Zhou YC, Li XP, Yu H, Guan JW. Rational design of secondary operation for penetrating head injury: A case report. Chinese Journal of Traumatology = Zhonghua Chuang Shang Za Zhi. 2020;**23**(2):84-88

[22] Anderson SA, Story PG. Case study of an orbital screwdriver injury. Journal of Ophthalmic Nursing & Technology. 1996;**15**(3):103-104

[23] Evans RJ, Richmond JM. An unusual death due to screwdriver impalement: A case report. The American Journal of Forensic Medicine and Pathology. 1996;**17**(1):70-72

[24] Ishikawa E, Meguro K, Yanaka K, Murakami T, Narushima K, Aoki T, et al. Intracerebellar penetrating injury and abscess due to a wooden foreign body--case report. Neurologia Medico-Chirurgica (Tokyo). 2000;**40**(9):458-462

[25] Schreckinger M, Orringer D, Thompson BG, La Marca F, Sagher O. Transorbital penetrating injury: Case series, review of the literature, and proposed management algorithm. Journal of Neurosurgery. 2011;**114**(1):53-61

[26] De Tommasi A, Cascardi P, De Tommasi C, Luzzi S, Ciappetta P. Emergency surgery in a severe penetrating skull base injury by a screwdriver: Case report and literature review. World Journal of Emergency Surgery: WJES. 2006;**1**:36

[27] Deveer M, Imamoglu F, Imamoglu C, Okten S. An incidental case of asymptomatic intracranial foreign body on CT. BML Case Reports. 10 Jun 2013;**2013**:bcr2013010230

[28] Hettige S, Kok K, Epaliyanage P, Thomas NW. Chopstick injury penetrating the skull base: A case report. Skull Base. 2010;**20**(3):219-222

[29] Maruya J, Yamamoto K, Wakai M, Kaneko U. Brain abscess following transorbital penetrating injury due to bamboo fragments--case report. Neurologia Medico-Chirurgica (Tokyo). 2002;**42**(3):143-146

[30] Encarnacion-Ramirez MJ, Aquino AA, Castillo REB, Melo-Guzman G, Lopez-Vujnovic D, Blas A, et al. Surgical management of a penetrating drill bit injury to the skull base. Surgical Neurology International. 2022;**13**:49

[31] Bajaj J, Agrawal M, Sinha VD. Blunt orbital injury causing traumatic intracranial aneurysm in a child. Journal of Neurosciences in Rural Practice. 2016;7(1):187-189

[32] Edem BE, Adekwu A, Efu ME, Kuni J, Onuchukwu G, Ugwuadu J. Anaesthetic and surgical management of

airway penetrating injuries in children in resource-poor setting: Case reports. International Journal of Surgery Case Reports. 2017;**39**:119-122

[33] Clark WC, Muhlbauer MS, Watridge CB, Ray MW. Analysis of 76 civilian craniocerebral gunshot wounds. Journal of Neurosurgery. 1986;**65**(1):9-14

[34] Miller CF, Brodkey JS, Colombi BJ. The danger of intracranial wood. Surgical Neurology. 1977;7(2):95-103

[35] Yoshihara S, Baba S, Kanemaru A, Ichikawa T. Craniofacial penetration by a wooden stick. European Annals of Otorhinolaryngology, Head and Neck Diseases. 2019;**136**(5):393-395

[36] Nguyen HS, Oni-Orisan A, Doan N, Mueller W. Transnasal penetration of a ballpoint pen: Case report and review of literature. World Neurosurgery. 2016;**96**(611):e1-e10

[37] Tsao YH, Kao CH, Wang HW, Chin SC, Moe KS. Transorbital penetrating injury of paranasal sinuses and anterior skull base by a plastic chair glide: Management options of a foreign body in multiple anatomic compartments. Otolaryngology and Head and Neck Surgery. 2006;**134**(1):177-179

[38] Zilinskiene L, Idle MR, Colley S. Emergency radiology: Maxillofacial and skull-base trauma. Trauma. 2014;**16**(4):243-255

[39] Martin S, Raup GH, Cravens G, Arena-Marshall C. Management of embedded foreign body: Penetrating stab wound to the head. Journal of Trauma Nursing. 2009;**16**(2):82-86

[40] Zhang D, Chen J, Han K, Yu M, Hou L. Management of penetrating skull base injury: A single institutional experience and review of the literature. BioMed Research International. 2017;**2017**:2838167

[41] Dunn IF, Kim DH, Rubin PA, Blinder R, Gates J, Golby AJ. Orbitocranial wooden foreign body: A pre-, intra-, and postoperative chronicle: Case report. Neurosurgery. 2009;**65**(2):E383-E384. discussion E4

[42] Eidsness R, Coupal DJ, Kelly ME, Hattingh S. Traumatic orbital injury. The Journal of Trauma. 2007;**62**(5):1286-1287

[43] Hiraishi T, Tomikawa M, Kobayashi T, Kawaguchi T. Delayed brain abscess after penetrating transorbital injury. No Shinkei Geka. 2007;**35**(5):481-486

[44] Huggins AB, Evans JJ, Flanders AE, Rabinowitz MP. Goat horn-induced intracranial emphysema and orbital injury. Orbit. 2016;**35**(6):355-356

[45] Bernal-Sprekelsen M, Alobid I, Mullol J, Trobat F, Tomas-Barberan M. Closure of cerebrospinal fluid leaks prevents ascending bacterial meningitis. Rhinology. 2005;**43**(4):277-281

[46] Wormald PJ, McDonogh M. 'Bath-plug' technique for the endoscopic management of cerebrospinal fluid leaks. The Journal of Laryngology and Otology. 1997;**111**(11):1042-1046

[47] Kazim SF, Shamim MS, Tahir MZ, Enam SA, Waheed S. Management of penetrating brain injury. Journal of Emergencies, Trauma, and Shock. 2011;**4**(3):395-402

[48] Williams JR, Aghion DM, Doberstein CE, Cosgrove GR, Asaad WF. Penetrating brain injury after suicide attempt with speargun: Case study and review of literature. Frontiers in Neurology. 2014;**5**:113

[49] Gutierrez-Gonzalez R, Boto GR, Rivero-Garvia M, Perez-Zamarron A, Gomez G. Penetrating brain injury by drill bit. Clinical Neurology and Neurosurgery. 2008;**110**(2):207-210

[50] Benzel EC, Day WT, Kesterson L, Willis BK, Kessler CW, Modling D, et al. Civilian craniocerebral gunshot wounds. Neurosurgery. 1991;**29**(1):67-71; discussion –2

[51] Zhu RC, Yoshida MC, Kopp M, Lin N. Treatment of a self-inflicted intracranial nail gun injury. BML Case Reports. 2021;**14**(1):e237122

[52] Brandvold B, Levi L, Feinsod M, George ED. Penetrating craniocerebral injuries in the Israeli involvement in the Lebanese conflict, 1982-1985. Analysis of a less aggressive surgical approach. Journal of Neurosurgery. 1990;**72**(1):15-21

[53] Levi L, Borovich B, Guilburd JN, Grushkiewicz I, Lemberger A, Linn S, et al. Wartime neurosurgical experience in Lebanon, 1982-85. I: Penetrating craniocerebral injuries. Israel Journal of Medical Sciences. 1990;**26**(10):548-554

[54] Cho J, Kim JH, Hong SD. Complex anterior skullbase fracture caused by a bottle cap: A case report and review of the literature. Journal of Rhinology. 2016;**23**:49-54

[55] Nishio Y, Hayashi N, Hamada H, Hirashima Y, Endo S. A case of delayed brain abscess due to a retained intracranial wooden foreign body: A case report and review of the last 20 years. Acta Neurochirurgica. 2004;**146**(8):847-850

[56] Pease M, Marquez Y, Tuchman A, Markarian A, Zada G. Diagnosis and surgical management of traumatic cerebrospinal fluid oculorrhea: Case report and systematic review of the literature. Journal of Neurological Surgery Reports. 2013;**74**(1):57-66

[57] Part 2: Prognosis in penetrating brain injury. The Journal of Trauma. 2001;**51**(Suppl. 2):S44-S86

[58] Blankenship BA, Baxter AB, McKahn GM 2nd. Delayed cerebral artery pseudoaneurysm after nail gun injury. AJR. American Journal of Roentgenology. 1999;**172**(2):541-542

[59] Freeman BJ, Ainscow DA. Nail gun injury: An update. Injury. 1994;**25**(2):110-111

[60] Woodall MN, Alleyne CH Jr. Nail-gun head trauma: A comprehensive review of the literature. Journal of Trauma and Acute Care Surgery. 2012;**73**(4):993-996

Chapter 2

Transnasal Endoscopic Pituitary Surgery: Indications, Technique, and Complications

Nazik Abdullah, Haytham Osman, Honida Ibrahim, Khalid Elzein and Ali Awad

Abstract

Pituitary neoplasm is the commonest sellar pathology, where pituitary adenoma heads the list, it accounts for 25% of all intracranial neoplasm. Although it is a benign lesion in most cases is located in a complex region; adjacent to important structures: optic chiasm, internal carotid arteries, suprasellar cistern, and cavernous sinuses, it presents with a variety of clinical scenarios. The Sella is situated at the center of the skull base, this made surgical access *via* craniotomy very challenging and is associated with considerable morbidity. Transnasal endoscopic pituitary surgery (TEPS) evolved rapidly, almost replacing the craniotomy approach, because it is minimally invasive and gives direct sellar access with excellent visualization. On the other hand, the learning curve of TEPS requires meticulous training to acquire surgical skills. Indications of TEPS, technique, complications, their prevention, and management are described. The multidisciplinary approach in managing pituitary adenoma is addressed, where a team of an endocrinologist, neurosurgeon, otolaryngologist, ophthalmologist, anesthesiologist, and neuroradiologist decide on a management plan for patients. Other disciplines share management of certain cases that is Oncologist, ICU specialists, and obstetrician. Long term follow-up is required by endocrinologists whereas revision surgery is considered in some patients.

Keywords: pituitary adenoma, transnasal, endoscopic, surgery, skull base, reconstruction, nasoseptal flap, CSF

1. Introduction

The pituitary gland is situated at the center of the skull base, in a saddle-like bone, the Sella, a complex anatomical region with critical neurovascular structures adjacent. This gland has a vital physiological function by acting as the chief controller of all the endocrine glands in the body. The complex anatomy, physiology, and clinical presentation of pathology made the journey of patients with pituitary tumors very challenging. Treatment goals of pituitary tumors are to relieve pressure on surrounding important structures, normalize hormone levels, and improve neurological deficits.

Options of treatment include surgery, medical therapy, radiation therapy, or a combination in an individualized patient's approach. Treatment choice depends on hormonal status, tumor size, type, and extension.

According to authors' experience, the decision of management plan, which includes the diagnosis, treatment, perioperative care, and follow is being taken by a dedicated formal multidisciplinary team, the team includes members from each of the following departments, endocrinology, neurosurgery, ophthalmology, otolaryngology, radiology, anesthesia/ICU and oncology. This team was created in the year 2017, and the importance of this team approach is thoroughly addressed later, in summary, it optimizes treatment options, improves the outcome of surgery, and reduces the complications rate.

Transnasal endoscopic pituitary surgery (TEPS) is an evolutionary approach to the management of pituitary tumors. This approach is minimally invasive, it utilizes the endoscope transnasally, without the requirement of external scalp incision and craniotomy. The endoscope allows for better visualization of the surgical field and consequently precise, safe, and effective surgical resection.

This procedure requires extensive knowledge of normal anatomy and anatomical variations, meticulous training, and surgical auditing to catch the learning curve. To master the skills of this surgery, both baseline training and continuous lifelong learning are required, these include hands-on cadaveric dissection and training on simulation models. The authors started endoscopic pituitary surgery in a center of excellence after creating a multidisciplinary team in 2017, bearing in mind that it is in a low-resource country and a limited facility center, and despite the unavailability of neuronavigation as routine, the outcome of surgery is satisfactory and improving, the complications are becoming less and more complicated cases are being operated. The surgeons, both neurosurgeons and otolaryngologists, were already well trained in endoscopic surgery with a wealthy experience before commencing pituitary endoscopic surgery.

The authors have experience of very advanced pathology with massive extension and late presentation of patients, the majority present with impaired vision, being referred from the ophthalmology department rather than the general practitioner, due to limited access to primary health services and delayed referrals. This puts a further burden on the team, particularly with the limited facilities. The authors' experience is unique, dealing with advanced cases with limited facilities, yet a reasonable outcome, implementing the "Do more with less" strategy.

2. Anatomy of the sella and suprasellar region

2.1 Anatomy of the sellar region

The anatomy of the gland has important clinical and surgical implications. The pituitary gland is situated in the pituitary fossa, also named the hypophyseal fossa or the sella turcica, a bony saddle as the name indicates in Latin. This bony saddle is located at the center of the skull base, it is fibro-osseous. The roof of the sphenoid sinus forms the floor of the pituitary fossa, this is demonstrated in the CT scan in **Figure 1** The sella turcica is bounded by bone, anteriorly, inferiorly, and posteriorly. The pituitary fossa is roofed by the diaphragma sellae, a dural fold with a central aperture; covering the fossa incompletely, *via* this central aperture passes the pituitary stalk with its' blood vessels.

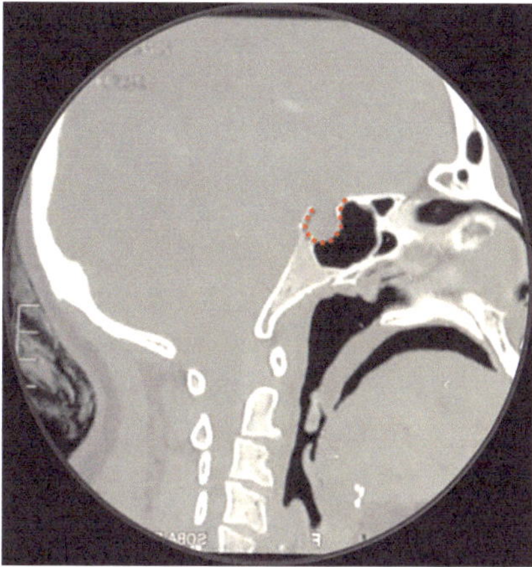

Figure 1.
Ct scan, sagittal cut, demonstrating the bony outlines, dashed red line, of the Sella turcica.

Laterally, the cavernous sinus is separated from the pituitary gland by a dural fold that forms the medial wall of the cavernous sinus. Antero-superiorly lies the optic chiasm, separated from the pituitary gland by the diaphragma sellae [1–3].

2.2 Variations of pituitary gland and sellar region

Variations of the gland should be taken into consideration when planning surgery, they may lengthen duration of resection, and some are dangerous leading to life-threatening complications [4].

The weight of the gland is variable according to gender. During pregnancy, the gland's weight increases and even doubles. The shape of the gland can be altered by pressure of the internal carotid arteries, leading to flattening of the pituitary gland. There is variation in the height of the gland, it ranges from 3 to 11 mm. When the gland does not fill the hypophyseal fossa, the suprasellar arachnoid cistern descends and encroaches on the fossa, in this case, it becomes a sellar component. The distance between the optic chiasm and the tuberculum sellae is very variable, it ranges between 1.5 to 8 mm. The sphenoid sinus is located on sellar floor, its extent of pneumatization is crucial in the accessibility of the sella during surgery when the transnasal approach is used [4].

A sellar type, where the sphenoid pneumatization extends well around the sellar floor is favorable for a transnasal approach as demonstrated in **Figure 2**, contrary to the conchal type, where access to sellar floor is difficult due to thick bone, in this case, image guide radiology is helpful to prevent complications, e.g., unintentional injury of important neighboring structures.

2.3 Parasellar and suprasellar anatomy

The cavernous sinus and the suprasellar cistern encompass the parasellar region. The lateral walls of the pituitary fossa are made up of dura mater, and it contains the cavernous sinus. The cavernous sinus consists of the internal carotid artery, sympathetic fibers, and cranial nerves III, IV, V, and VI. The suprasellar cistern encompasses the optic chiasm, part of the third ventricle, the hypothalamus, and the tuber cinereum [2, 5].

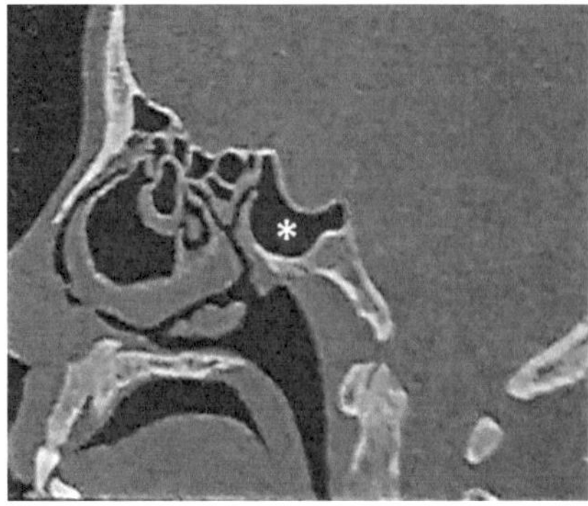

Figure 2.
CT scan, sagittal cut, demonstrating a sellar pneumatization of sphenoid sinus (star), which is favorable for endoscopic transnasal endoscopic pituitary surgery (TEPS).

2.4 Blood supply of the pituitary gland

The pituitary gland is enriched with blood supply, it is a well-vascularized organ. The hypothalamo-hypophyseal portal system connects the blood supply of the gland with the hypothalamus. This connection is very important in regulating the secretory function of the gland, it will be discussed later in the physiology section.

The anterior lobe of the gland receives its blood supply from the superior hypophyseal artery, which originates either from the internal carotid artery or the posterior communicating artery. The posterior lobe of the gland receives its blood supply from the inferior hypophyseal artery which originates from the meningo-hypophyseal artery which is a branch of the internal carotid artery. The intermediate lobe receives blood from the capillaries of the anterior and posterior lobes. The pituitary stalk and parts of the optic nerve and chiasm are supplied by branches from the superior hypophyseal artery. A primary plexus is formed from the internal carotid artery and the posterior communicating artery, it supplies the median eminence, and the hypothalamic cells end at the median eminence, hence the primary plexus receives regulatory factors. Capillaries from all lobes form venules, these venules form the secondary plexus, and the latter drain into the cavernous sinus *via* the portal hypophyseal veins [6, 7].

2.5 Histology of the pituitary gland

The pituitary gland is composed histologically of two parts, the adenohypophysis, and the neurohypophysis.

2.5.1 Adenohypophysis

It is a secretory part, responsible for hormone production and secretion. It is composed of well-defined acini, there are six cell lines, five of which are hormone-producing cell lines, namely: Somatotrophs, lactotrophs, corticotrophs, thyrotrophs, and gonadotrophs. The folliculostellate cells form the sixth cell line, which is a nonhormone-producing cell line.

The following structures make up the anterior pituitary gland:

Pars distalis, it forms most of the bulk of the anterior pituitary gland, it is composed of cells that produce hormones, arranged in the form of follicles of different sizes. Based on the staining characteristics, the hormone-producing cells are classified as:

Acidophils: The cytoplasm stains red, they are composed of polypeptide hormones. Soamtptrophs and lactotrophs are acidophils.

Basophils: The cytoplasm stains blue to purple, they are composed of glycoproteins, thyrotrophs, gonadotrophs, and corticotrophs are basophils.

Chromophobes: As the name states, they do not stain. Stem cells that are yet to differentiate into hormone-producing cells form this cell line.

Pars Tuberalis: The tubular stalk has anterior and posterior parts. It encircles the infundibular stem. The infundubular stem is composed of unmyelinated axons, that originate from the hypothalamic nuclei. Two hormones accumulate in these axons; oxytocin and vasopressin, in the form of ovoid eosinophilic swellings along the stem of the infundibulum. They make the herring bodies.

Pars intermedia: It is located between the pars distalis and the posterior pituitary gland. Follicles containing a colloid matrix form the pars intermedia, it includes the reminder of Rathke's pouch cleft. Melanocyte-stimulating hormones and endorphins are produced by these cells.

The initial primary signal hormones are synthesized in the hypothalamus to stimulate the pituitary gland. Production of these primary signal hormones is in the cell body of the neurons, the axons project to end at the gland in the fenestrated portal capillaries. They are then carried *via* the blood stream to reach the pituitary gland, where specific cells are stimulated or inhibited [1].

2.5.2 Neurohypophysis

This is a specialized neuroendocrine structure.

It is composed of both, pars nervosa and the infundibular stalk. The axons that originate in the hypothalamus, form the neurohypophysis. These axons are encircled by glial cells called the pituicytes. The pituicytes have elongated processes that run along with the axons. The axons form the hypothalamo-hypophyseal tract, which terminates near the posterior lobe sinusoids [1].

2.6 Embryology of the pituitary gland

Two different origins form the pituitary gland. The adenohypophysis is derived from the oral ectoderm. The neurohypophysis is derived from neural ectoderm. The posterior lobe is derived as an extension of the central nervous system (third ventricle neural primordia) [3].

3. Physiology of the pituitary gland

The following are the hormones produced and secreted from the anterior pituitary: Adrenocorticotropic Hormone (ACTH), Prolactin (PRL), Luteinizing Hormone (LH) and Follicle-Stimulating Hormone (FSH), Growth Hormone or Somatotropin (GH) and Thyroid Stimulating Hormone (TSH) [6, 8–10]. Two hormones are released from the posterior pituitary: Oxytocin and Arginine Vasopressin (AVP) or Antidiuretic Hormone (ADH) [9, 11–13].

4. Pathology

Endocrine and neurological disorders are encountered in the sellar region, due to neoplasms arising from the adenohypophysis, such as pituitary adenoma, which heads the list ardently, it is associated with excessive hormonal production, examples are acromegaly and Cushing's disease, other pathologies include cysts or tumors derived from remnants of Rathke's pouch (Rathke's cleft cyst, craniopharyngioma), tumors derived from the neurohypophysis and pituitary stalk (pituicytoma and granular cell tumor) and tumors of the parasellar bone (chordoma). Further, conditions such as lymphocytic or granulomatous hypophysitis, present clinically like tumors [3].

Pituitary adenomas are common intracranial tumors, they are benign clonal neoplasms, originating from the endocrine epithelial cells of the adenohypophysis. Adenoma of the pituitary gland has a wide spectrum of presentation, in 22%, it is clinically silent and discovered accidentally on MRI scans of the brain, around 14% are autopsy finding, and It accounts for 25% of clinically apparent intracranial tumors [3, 4].

Pituitary adenoma in common with other adenomas of endocrine origin, share the following characteristics: round nuclei with finely dispersed chromatin, distinct multiple nucleoli, and granular cytoplasm. They express both markers of neurosecretory granules and epithelial differentiation. Wide morphological features of pituitary adenoma are described based on hormonal, or genetic subtype, or due to treatment effect. Pituitary adenoma is a benign neoplasm, but it can be locally invasive and destructive. Excess hormone secretion gives rise to metabolic disorders that render it malignant on a clinical basis [3].

4.1 WHO classification

According to the following factors, pituitary adenomas are classified: size, clinically silent or functional, hormone or cytokeratin expression profile, histologic features, or somatic mutations. Markers of cytodifferentiation are the principal classifiers in the 2004 edition of the WHO classification of endocrine tumors. Adenoma is further categorized into typical pituitary adenoma, pituitary carcinoma, and atypical pituitary adenoma [14]. The criteria of atypia are subjective, and the clinical significance is ill-defined, this warrants the need for longitudinal studies to label atypia [15]. The current 2004 classification is described in **Table 1** [16–18].

Adenoma type	Transcription Factors	Hormones	Cytokeratin
GH-producing adenomas			
Densely granulated somatotroph adenoma	Pit-1	GH, a-SU	diffuse
Sparsely granulated somatotroph adenoma	Pit-1	GH	dot-like
Mammosomatotroph adenoma	Pit-1, ER	GH, PRL, a-SU	diffuse
Mixed somatotroph and lactotroph andenoma	Pit-1, ER	GH, PRL, a-SU	diffuse
PRL-producing adenomas			
Sparsely granulated lactotroph adenoma	Pit-1, ER	PRL (Golgi)	diffuse
Densely granulated lactotroph adenoma	Pit-1, ER	PRL (diffuse)	diffuse
Acidophil stem-cell adenoma	Pit-1, ER	PRL (diffuse), GH	rare dot-like
TSH-producing adenoma			
Thyrotroph adenoma	Pit-1, GATA-2	b-TSH, a-SU	diffuse
ACTH-producing adenomas			
Densely granulated corticotroph adenoma	Tpit	ACTH	diffuse

DOI: http://dx.doi.org/10.5772/intechopen.1003030

Adenoma type	Transcription Factors	Hormones	Cytokeratin
Sparsely granulated corticotroph adenoma	Tpit	ACTH	diffuse
Crooke's cell adenoma	Tpit	ACTH	ring-like
Gonadotropin-producing adenoma			
Gonadotroph adenoma	SF-1, GATA-2, ER	b-FSH, b-LH, a-SU	diffuse
Plurihormonal adenomas			
Silent type III adenoma	Pit-1 (?), ER	Multiple	diffuse
Unusual plurihormonal adenoma (NOS)	multiple	Multiple	n/a
Hormone negative adenoma			
Null cell adenoma	None	None	diffuse

Table 1.
Classification according to side is described as follows: Microadenomas (<10 mm) which are often within the Sella turcica, macroadenomas (≥10 mm) which may be contained in the Sella turcica but also infiltrate into the superior, inferior, and or lateral extrasellar space, and giant adenomas (≥40 mm).

5. Symptoms and signs

The presentation of pituitary adenoma depends on tumor size and functional status [19, 20].

Pituitary microadenoma (less than 1 cm) is usually an incidental finding on MRI Brain and patients are asymptomatic unless the tumor is hormonally active, while pituitary macroadenoma (more than 1 cm) presents with symptoms and signs of space-occupying lesion in addition to hormonal deficiency or hormonal excess. Pituitary apoplexy is a complicated adenoma, where sudden hemorrhage ensues into the adenoma, it presents with severe headache and acute vision changes besides mass effect.

5.1 Symptoms from mass effect (nonfunctioning adenoma)

5.1.1 Visual impairment

Vision changes occur in 40–60% of patients. It presents as bitemporal defect in most cases, followed by homonymous defect and diplopia. Suprasellar extension of large pituitary tumors compress the optic chiasm leading to the previously mentioned visual field defects and impaired acuity, while Involvement of cranial nerves by invasive tumors explains diplopia and blindness [21, 22].

5.1.2 Headache

Headache is commonly reported in pituitary adenoma; however, it is a non-specific symptom [22]. It is of sudden onset and severe in apoplexy as mentioned earlier.

5.1.3 Hormonal deficiency

Patients with pituitary adenoma may present with hormonal deficiencies, where one or more hormones of the anterior pituitary are deficient. In gonadotrophin deficiency, females present with amenorrhea, and males present with erectile dysfunction. Growth hormone (GH) when deficient in adults, presents with fatigue and weight loss. Thyroid Stimulating Hormone deficiency (TSH) leads to weight gain, fatigue, constipation, and cold intolerance. Symptoms of Adrenal Cortical Stimulating Hormone (ACTH) deficiency are those of hypoadrenalism; fatigue, weight loss, arthralgia, dizziness, nausea, low blood pressure, and abdominal pain.

5.1.4 Case scenario no (1)

A 44-year-old male, with no significant past medical history, presented to the ER with a history of sudden loss of vision for 1 day preceded by severe headache. No history of loss of consciousness. Examination revealed a fully oriented person with intact higher functions, he was totally blind (fundus examination revealed papilledema grade 4). Investigations: Hormonal profile showed features of panhypopituitarism. Brain MRI showed sellar lesion with suprasellar extension. Clinically and radiologically, the diagnosis of apoplexy was made. Intraoperatively soft tumor tissues were retrieved with hematoma and infarcted debris as in **Figures 3–6**. Marked improvement of vision was acheived, immediately postoperatively.

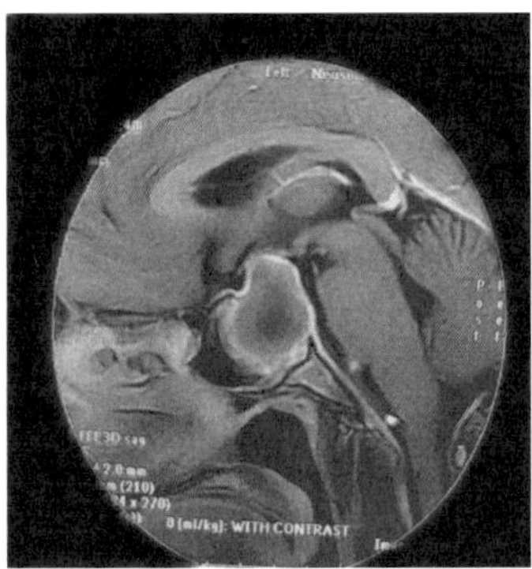

Figure 3.
MRI, sagittal view, showing a mixed signal intensity macroadenoma.

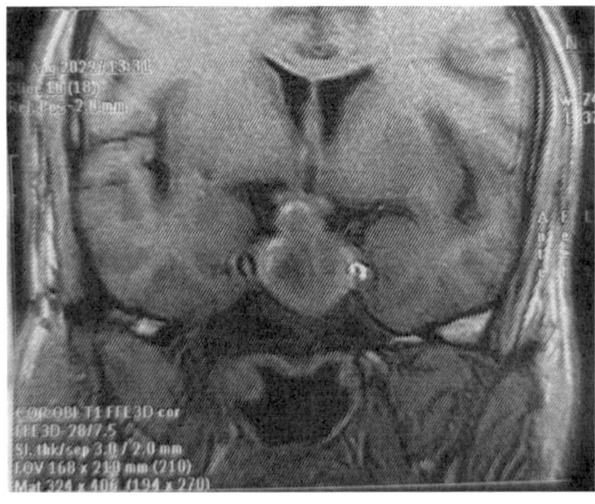

Figure 4.
MRI coronal view of macroadenoma with different signal intensity, suggesting hemorrhage (apoplexy).

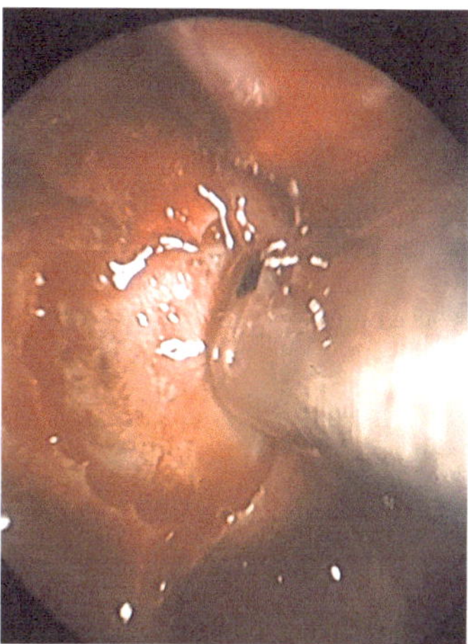

Figure 5.
Endoscopic view, showing adequate sphenoidotomy, drilled sellar floor, and dura exposed.

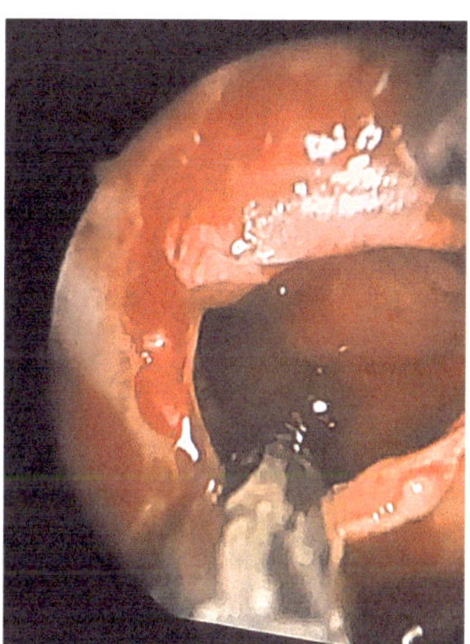

Figure 6.
Tumor cavity, gross tumor resection, with decompression of adjacent carotids, cistern, and optic chiasm, note suprasellar cistern at 12 O'Clock.

5.2 Symptoms of functioning adenomas

Patients with secreting adenomas present according to the hormone being excessively produced, the following clinical scenarios are observed:

5.2.1 Prolactin-secreting adenomas

High levels of prolactin suppress the gonadotrophin levels leading to infertility, osteoporosis, and decreased libido in males and females. Males present with gynecomastia and erectile dysfunction and females present with amenorrhea and galactorrhea.

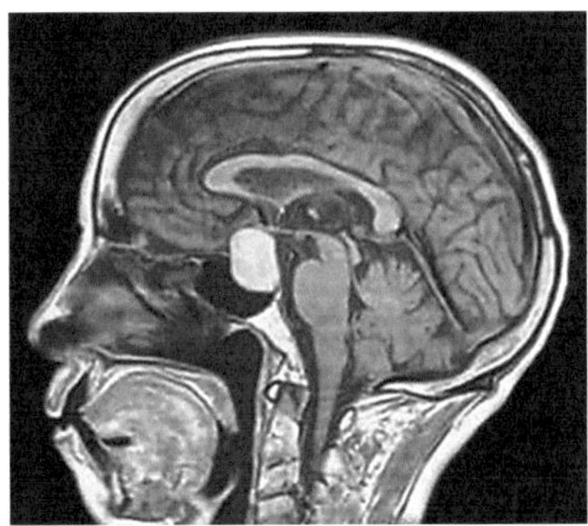

Figure 7.
MRI, TI, sagittal view demonstrating macroadenoma.

5.2.2 GH-secreting adenoma (acromegaly)

Patients complain of headaches, vision changes, and an increase in ring size and shoe size, others present with carpal tunnel syndrome and excessive sweating. On examination, they have coarse facial features, frontal bossing, enlarged nose, protruded mandible, and an enlarged tongue. Hypertension, cardiomyopathy, multiple colonic polyps, and obstructive sleep apnea are comorbidities.

5.2.3 ACTH-secreting adenoma (Cushing's disease)

Weight gain is the chief complaint, others include muscle weakness, mood disorders, easy bruising, and multiple fractures. Clinically, patients have moon face, supraclavicular fat, ecchymoses, and striae on armpits and abdomen.

5.2.4 TSH secreting adenoma

Patients present with palpitations, weight loss, heat intolerance, and arrythmias. A goiter and tremors are usually obvious features.

5.2.5 Case scenario No (2)

A 39-year-old lady presented with features of acromegaly and secondary infertility, no other symptoms, hormone profile revealed an elevated growth hormone level. MRI showed pituitary macroadenoma as in **Figure** 7, transnasal endoscopic pituitary surgery was performed. This lady showed obvious improvement in acromegaly features, and she delivered a baby girl 1 year after surgery.

6. Radiological assessment of pituitary lesions

The image of choice of the pituitary gland is MR. Thin sections (1–2) mm are required to have detailed study of the sellar region, thin cuts are performed in both the coronal and sagittal planes. The mainstay of pituitary imaging is T1 weighted sequences, pre and post contrast [23]. Post contrast MR sequences in dynamic fashion (during the first minute) after contrast injection is of great benefit, as it maximizes the

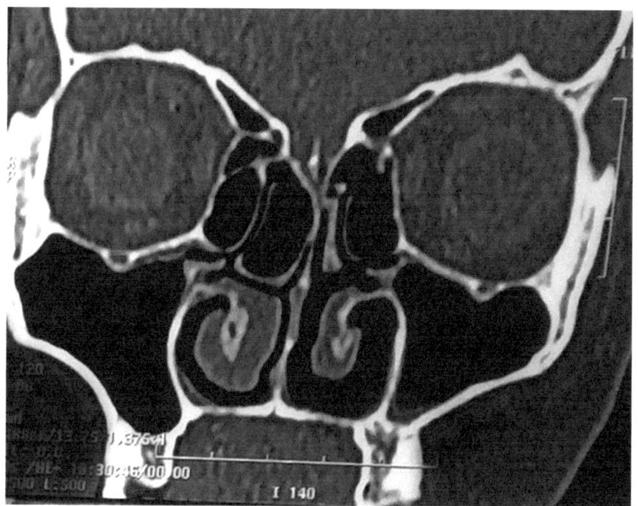

Figure 8.
Coronal CT scan of the nose and sinuses, showing bilateral concha bullosa. Note narrowing of the nasal cavity.

visibility of adenomas within the pituitary gland, which typically shows less enhancement than the normal pituitary tissue, this differential enhancement is best addressed within the first arterial phase of contrast injection. In the majority of pituitary adenomas, they are well demonstrated on a standard acquisition (non-dynamic) scan after contrast injection [24]. The high field strength 3 Tesla MR scanners, which are replacing the 1.5 Tesla machines, provide high-resolution pituitary images.

Excellent soft tissue characterization is well provided by MRI, in the contrary, CT does not provide this, but can be useful for investigation when MR is contraindicated or unavailable, or if identification of calcification around the sella is significantly required [25]. CT of the nose and sinuses is essential if surgery is indicated, where anatomical variations and sphenoid pneumatization are identified preoperatively. **Figure 8** demonstrates bilateral concha bullosa.

7. Treatment and management

Management of pituitary tumors requires a team approach with participation from the following departments: Internal medicine, endocrinology, ophthalmology, radiology, neurosurgery, ENT, and anesthesia/ICU. A specialized neuroradiologist is an important team member as MRI needs to be done with the pituitary protocol.

7.1 Treatment of non-functioning adenomas

Surgery is indicated in the presence of one or more of the following conditions [26]:

- Vision change, for example, visual field defect, ophthalmoplegia, and sudden vision loss

- Compression of the optic nerve or optic chiasm on imaging

- Pituitary apoplexy with visual disturbances
- Hypopituitarism
- Significant growth of pituitary tumor over time

Pituitary adenomas, when less than 1 cm is labeled as microadenomas, although there is no clinical significance of this threshold, a cut-off of 20 or 30 mm is demonstrated to be more relevant, therefore more studies are needed to examine the significance of classification according to size, and probably to reset a cut-off size. One study concluded that there was no difference in the rate of surgery or survival for pituitary adenomas in the range of 30–50 mm, questioning the 4-mm cut-off threshold for labeling giant pituitary adenoma [27].

Surgery is aimed at improvement in visual symptoms and improvement of hormonal dysfunction. Most patients improve. Radiotherapy is a choice for patients with persistent or residual tumors.

Annual follow-up is required for nonfunctional adenomas that do not require surgery, endocrinological and radiological follow-ups (by MR,) are performed to assess the development of hypopituitarism and tumor growth.

7.2 Treatment of individual functioning tumors

7.2.1 Prolactin secreting adenomas

The first line of treatment for prolactin-secreting tumors is Dopamine Agonists (DA) e.g. Cabergoline and bromocriptine. Cabergoline controls prolactin secretion in more than 90% of tumors. Tumors regress in size accordingly, and when there is no longer tumor in the MRI, cabergoline is discontinued after 2 years. Annual monitoring of prolactin levels is required to detect recurrence after stopping cabergoline. Prolactin-secreting tumors that are resistant to cabergoline are treated by surgical resection. Other indications of surgery are the development of adverse effects of dopamine agonists that require cessation, patients who desire pregnancy, and tumors more than 1 cm.

When medications and frequent surgery fail to control tumor size, prolactinoma is then labeled as aggressive, in this case, radiotherapy is indicated.

7.2.2 GH secreting adenomas

Surgery is the first line for GH-secreting adenoma. Surgery is effective in 80–90% of microadenoma and in 40–60% of macroadenoma. Medical treatment (somatostatin analog) is offered for patients with persistently elevated levels of growth hormone after surgery and for inoperable invasive tumors.

Radiation therapy, although lately effective, is deferred for patients with elevated GH after surgery.

7.2.3 ACTH secreting adenoma

Cortisol levels are reduced rapidly by surgical resection of pituitary tumors. This is the first line of treatment for Cushing's disease, surgery is effective in 70–90% of patients. Although bilateral adrenalectomy is effective in leading to immediate relief of hypercortisolemia, it results in adrenal insufficiency, which requires lifelong supplements.

Medications that reduce ACTH secretion are cabergoline and SSA (pasireotide, pasireotide LAR). Others include ketoconazole, metyrapone, mitotane and etomidate. Mifepristone is a glucocorticoid blocker used in selected cases.

Radiotherapy is an adjuvant after surgery and medical treatment.

7.2.4 TSH secreting adenoma

The first line of treatment is pituitary surgery with a 50–90% cure rate. Hyperthyroidism is controlled before surgery to avoid a thyroid storm. Patients who are not cured by surgery can be treated with SSA to decrease both TSH levels and tumor size, failure of SSA implies its combination with radiation therapy [26].

8. Preoperative preparation and interprofessional team approach

Patients with pituitary tumors require a combined approach and coordination between the endocrinologist, the neurosurgeon, the ophthalmologist, the ENT surgeon, and the anesthesiologist.

Surgical outcome depends on preoperative status and assessment, intraoperative events, and postoperative complications therefore, patients' counseling is very important; the expectations and anticipated complications should be discussed and explained to the patient clearly, in this regard the input from each department is crucial.

Preoperative routine tests include complete blood count, electrolytes, liver function test, urine analysis, and coagulation profile. Endocrine assessment by assay of pituitary hormones and hormones of related glands are included. N.B. women with amenorrhea should always have a pregnancy test. Any preoperative manifestations of diseases secondary to pituitary dysfunction must be controlled.

Abnormal thyroid function test and adrenal gland dysfunction must be detected preoperatively, and normalized. Hydrocortisone is administered only to patients with low levels of corticoids as a replacement. Comorbidities associated with acromegaly and Cushing's disease should be evaluated thoroughly.

MRI head with pituitary protocol, CT scan of the nose and sinuses with nasal endoscopy by ENT surgeon are prerequisite for surgery. A swab from the nasopharynx is taken for bacteriology study to confirm pathogen-free nasal mucosa. Optimal intraoperative management depends on the indication for surgery and patient's disease. The advantage of rapid emergence from anesthesia is that it allows for early neurologic assessment, where common and serious surgical complications are identified [28].

9. Anesthetic management

Maintenance of hemodynamic stability, adequate cerebral perfusion and oxygenation, appropriate position of the patient, excellent surgical exposure, and quick recovery from anesthesia to assess neurological signs are the main goals of anesthetic management [14, 29].

A pharyngeal pack is placed after endotracheal intubation to prevent aspiration and filling of the stomach with debris, this will reduce post-operative nausea and vomiting. Local anesthetic application and vasopressin to the mucosal surfaces result in systemic hypertension and cardiac arrhythmia. These are transient effects and are treated with short-acting medications. Myocardial ischemia has been reported when vasoconstrictors are used excessively.

Fixation of endotracheal tube is very important, to prevent dislodgement as endotracheal tube is inaccessible during the operation.

Compression stockings are of paramount importance to prevent deep vein thrombosis with consequent pulmonary embolism.

Regarding the choice of anesthetic agents, it is like intracranial surgeries, and it depends on the patient's comorbidities.

10. Surgical treatment of pituitary tumors

10.1 Surgical approaches for pituitary tumors and patient selection

Surgery of the pituitary gland evolved from transcranial approach to transnasal transsphenoid approaches, either using the microscope or the endoscope [30, 31].

Fibrous tumors, failure of transsphenoidal resection, and dumbbell tumors that pass *via* a very narrow diaphragma sellae aperture are indications for transcranial approach.

The transcranial approach is claimed to have a greater visual improvement for long-term pituitary adenomas, nevertheless, it has a greater risk of postoperative pituitary dysfunction [32–34].

10.2 The learning curve

Transnasal endoscopic pituitary surgery (TEPS) has a learning curve like every other surgical technique. Results are not satisfactory at the beginning of the learning curve, however after achieving this curve the complications are reduced significantly. To master endoscopic pituitary surgery a range of 17–50 surgeries are required [35, 36].

Operative time decreases significantly in simple tumors; complex operations would have a longer learning curve. Similarly the gross tumor resection (GTR) rate, shows a gradual and continuous learning process [37].

Attending workshops, hands-on cadaveric dissection, practice on models, and observation of live surgeries are essential for skills acquisition. A training model using a skull and eggs is useful to improve surgical techniques in TEPS [38].

10.3 Patient selection

For a beginner surgeon, favorable cases are started with. The criteria for selecting patients are nonfunctioning adenoma, tumors confined to the sella without supra or parasellar extension, and a well-pneumatized sphenoid sinus. Unfavorable factors are extensive tumors with parasellar or suprasellar extension, dumbbell tumors, recurrent tumors, conchal/presellar sphenoid sinus, and associated acromegaly or Cushing's disease.

DOI: http://dx.doi.org/10.5772/intechopen.1003030

10.4 Preoperative radiological study and planning

MRI with pituitary protocol and CT of the nose, sinuses, and skull base are basic radiological investigations.

Checklist for radiological assessment [39]:

1. Size of nasal airway; it is jeopardized by deviated nasal septum and concha bullosa.

2. Anatomy of paranasal sinuses; extent of pneumatization, intra/inter-sphenoid septa, Onodi cell or concha bullosa.

3. Presence of sinus infection, as this delays pituitary surgery until it is cleared medically or surgically.

4. Anatomy of the sella; bony defects, anatomical variations, and abnormal carotid anatomy.

5. If the tumor is hypointense in T1, it is more likely to be firm in consistency.

6. Size of the tumor, a giant tumor may require an additional craniotomy approach or the presence of hydrocephalus as in **Figure 9**.

7. Extension of the tumor-like suprasellar and para sellar involvement, involvement of nearby structures, and encasement of carotid artery or invasion of cavernous sinus

8. Identification of the normal pituitary gland.

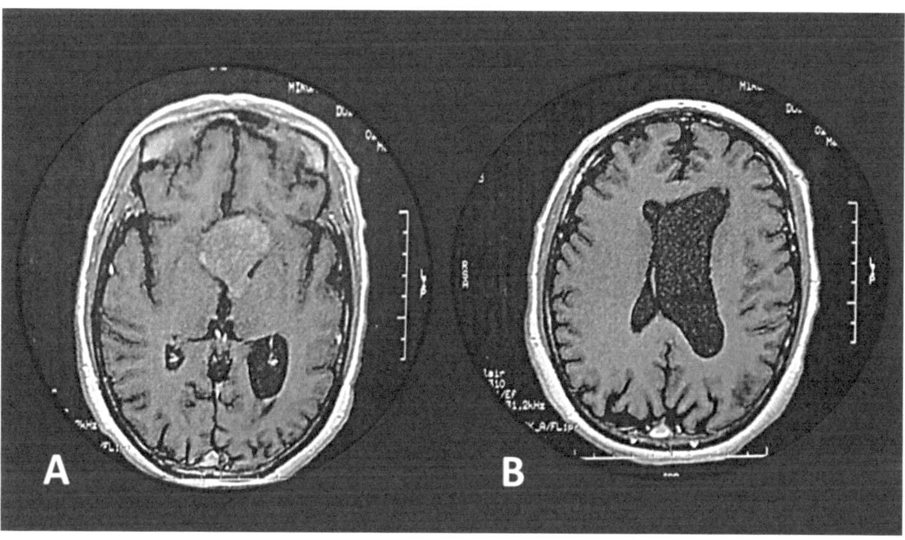

Figure 9.
MRI brain T1, Giant pituitary adenoma with suprasellar extension in (A), causing obstructive hydrocephalus as in (B).

9. Radiological features of apoplexy

10. Optic chiasm identification

11. Pituitary stalk deviation

10.5 Surgical stages

Surgery is divided into 4 stages: Nasal, sphenoid, sellar, and reconstruction stages as demonstrated briefly in the surgical video.

10.6 Operative room setup, equipment, and endoscopes

The operation room should be spacious to accommodate the necessary equipment, instruments, and personnel. The operating room plan is shown in **Figure 10**.

In nasal sphenoid and reconstruction stages, the main surgeon is on right side of the patient. The second surgeon; one on the right side of the surgeon and the third surgeon across the patient. In sellar stage, the main surgeon exchanges position with the second surgeon as shown in **Figure 11**, the latter holds the endoscope to allow for three and/or four hands technique.

It is essential to supply the operative room with an appropriate surgical instrumentation, to optimize the different stages of the operation. Equipment should include an up-to-date endoscopic unit; A high definition resolution screen adds to accuracy in visualization and hence precision in surgery, an image-guided monitor, set for endoscopic nasal surgery, Cappabianca set for skull base and pituitary surgery, and powered instruments; micro-debrider and a high-speed drill. Bipolar suction diathermy is an important surgical tool as it provides a bloodless surgical field with good visualization.

Different degrees of endoscopes add to surgical field revelation, the sheath makes the surgeon's grip more stable, and the irrigation system lessens the in-and-out movement of

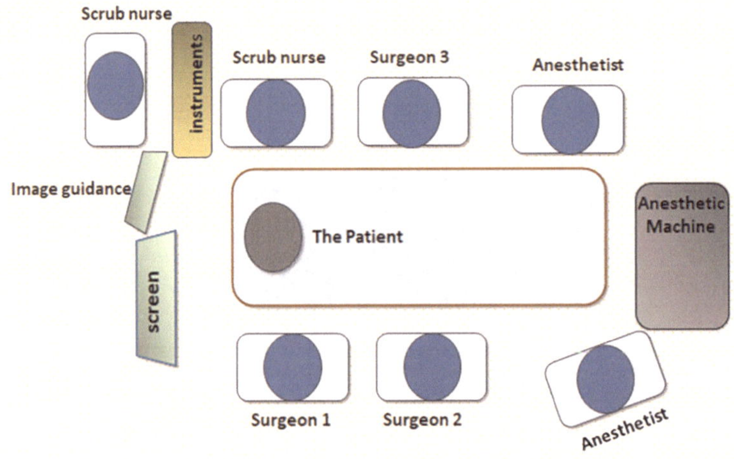

Figure 10.
Diagram of operating room arrangement of equipment, instruments and personnel for transnasal endoscopic pituitary surgery, during nasal, sphenoid and reconstruction stages.

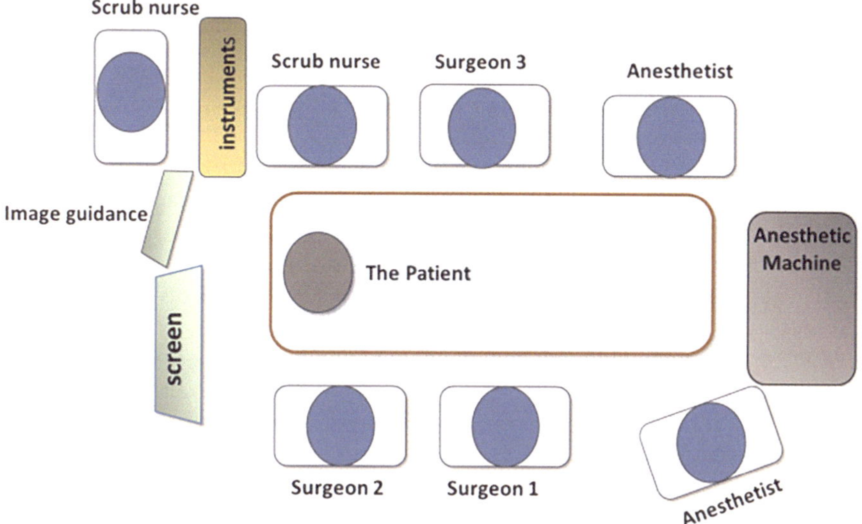

Figure 11.
Diagram of operating room arrangement of equipment, instruments and personnel for transnasal endoscopic pituitary surgery, during sellar stage.

Surgical stage	Endoscope	Instrument
Nasal stage & Sphenoid stage	Endoscope 0°, Length 18 cm, Diameter 4 mm, 5 mm External sheath and irrigation system and anti-fog	Nasal endoscopy set Micro-debrider High speed Drill Bipolar diathermy ± Navigation probe
Sellar stage	Endoscope 0°, 30°, 45°, Length 18, 30 cm Diameter 4 mm, 2.7 mm External sheath and irrigation system and anti-fog ± Reversed Endoscope version	Cappabianca set Bipolar diathermy ± Navigation probe
Reconstruction Stage	Endoscope 0°, Length 18 cm, Diameter 4 mm External sheath and irrigation system and anti-fog	Nasal endoscopy set

Table 2.
Summary of instruments required for different surgical stages.

the endoscope for cleaning. Cappabianca set is a set of instruments designed for endoscopic skull base and pituitary surgery, the instruments are longer than nasal surgery pieces, and unlike the bayonet for microscopic surgery are straight [40, 41]. Summary of instruments required for each stage is presented in **Table 2**. Image guidance is very important intraoperatively, when there are nasal anatomical variations like Onodi cell, deviated nasal septum, conchal or presellar sphenoid, kissing carotids and in revision surgery. In most of the centers it is a routine adjunct during surgery.

10.7 Positioning and scrubbing

The authors advise instillation of decongestant nasal drops (oxymetazoline) 7 days before surgery, three times a day.

It is recommended by some surgeons to be used the night before surgery and the day of surgery before taking the patient to the theater [14].

The position of the patient on operating table is supine in the reverse Trendelenburg position, hips and knees are slightly flexed, and the trunk is elevated 20 degrees [14]. Head of the patient is neutral, with a horse shoe head holder. The bridge of the nose is horizontal, parallel to the floor, and the head is turned 15 degrees toward the surgeon. When neuronavigation is used a three pin head rest or a band are fixed [41, 42].

The endotracheal tube is fixed to the lower jaw at the left side, nasogastric tube is optional, it helps in aspiration of blood and secretions before endotracheal tube extubation.

Lumbar drain may be inserted in patients having a large tumor with a considerable suprasellar extension, but this is not routine with controversy [39]. No lumbar drain was inserted for any of the patients operated by the authors.

A urine catheter is mandatory to monitor output, not only during surgery, but more significantly during the postoperative period to diagnose diabetes insipidus.

For antisepsis, betadine-soaked cotton patties are inserted in nasal cavities after positioning of the patient [39].

The patient is then draped leaving only the nostrils exposed, Suction tubes and cables including camera, light and irrigation cables are tied and placed on the left side of the patient or on a table to have a free surgical field.

Surgical stages description:

10.7.1 Nasal stage

Endoscopic examination of the nose is performed using 0 degree endoscope, usually insertion of the endoscope at the level of the floor is limited by the enlarged head of inferior turbinate (IT).

Decongestion of the inferior turbinate is done by insertion of cotton patties immersed in diluted adrenaline solution 1 in 200,000 and or oxymetazoline, sometimes infusion with diluted adrenaline solution 1 in 500,000 is required in grossly enlarged IT, in the latter case, inhalation of anesthetic like halothane if in use, should be withdrawn to prevent occurrence of arrythmia.

Landmarks are ascertained on endoscopic examination of the nose bilaterally, these are inferior turbinate, middle turbinate, choana, eustachian tube, vomer, and sphenoid sinus ostium.

In most cases, out fracture of middle turbinate is required for visualization and instrumentation, it is pushed by a blunt dissector laterally against its' second part preserving the mucosa and avoiding a flail (hypermobile) middle turbinate, if this happened partial resection of the lower half of it is advised while keeping the axilla intact.

Natural ostium of sphenoid sinus is located between superior turbinate and nasal septum, occasionally a supreme turbinate is present, in this case, the ostium lies between the supreme turbinate and nasal septum, it is apparent in most cases, seldomly not obvious, where gentle probing at its expected site reveals it. To double check the sphenoid sinus ostium, it is approximately 1.1–1.5 cm above choanal arch. The navigation is very helpful in certain anatomical variants e.g. conchal and presellar sphenoid.

Harvesting a nasoseptal flap is performed as early as this stage. Identification of sphenoid sinus ostium is a prerequisite to fashioning this flap, it is

Pedicled on the nasoseptal artery, this artery is a branch of the posterior septal artery that branches from the sphenopalatine artery, the latter originates from the maxillary artery [43].

A standard flap is made up of two parallel lines, the inferior line is over the maxillary crest and the superior line is 1–2 cm below the superior aspect of the nasal septum to spare the olfactory epithelium. The two lines are joined anteriorly by a vertical incision. Posteriorly the two incisions are not parallel, they rather fan from the sphenoid sinus opening superiorly and from the arch of the choana inferiorly, in this fashion the pedicle of the flap is preserved with its' blood supply (NSA) [44]. It is illustrated in **Figure 12**.

The flap is composed of mucoperichondrium anteriorly and mucoperiosteum posteriorly. The nasoseptal artery crosses from the lateral nasal wall to the septum passing in a coronal line that is midway between lower lip of sphenoid sinus ostium and arch of the choana. A viable flap with intact blood supply requires both a subperiosteal and subperichondrial plane of dissection throughout the whole length of the flap, and an intact mucoperiosteum in the area between arch of the choana and sphenoid sinus ostium. A unilateral flap is elevated from the right side. In an accidental tear of the flap, a left flap can be harvested, one flap is adequate for reconstruction of the skull base in pituitary macroadenoma.

The flap is then placed in the nasopharynx and protected by a nasal pack that is placed inferiorly to occlude the choana, it is kept (stored) until the stage of reconstruction.

In the left nostril, middle turbinate is out fractured, and sphenoid sinus ostium is identified. A vertical incision is made on the posterior part of nasal septum with elevation of mucoperiosteum, the latter is removed by micro-debrider as far posterolateral as sphenoid sinus ostium, the vomer and face of sphenoid bone are exposed.

Posterior septectomy is then performed. The vomer is thin in females compared to males; a blunt dissector easily penetrates through and through, Posterior one-third of the nasal septum is removed by a backbiter to allow for bi-nostril instrumentation. By removal of the posterior part of vomer ends the nasal stage.

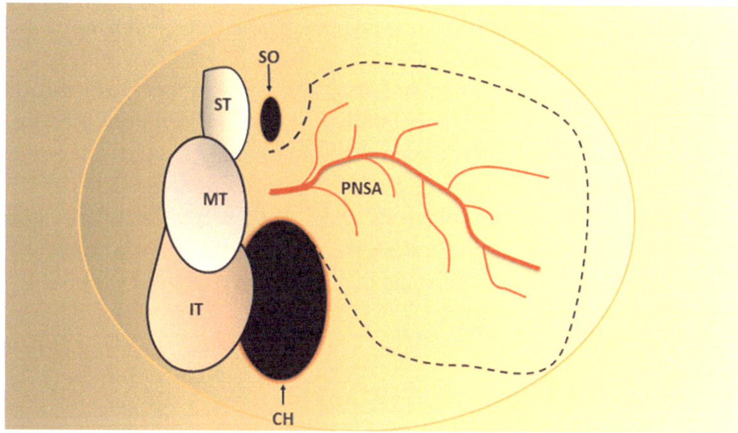

Figure 12.
IT: Inferior turbinate, MT: Middle turbinate, ST: Superior turbinate. SO: Sphenoid ostium, CH: Choana. PNSA: Posterior nasal septal artery. Posterior nasal septal artery passes in a subperiosteal plane mid-way between sphenoid sinus ostium and choanal arch. Dashed line demonstrates flap incision, note that it fans from posterior to anterior with a steep rise at upper incision line posteriorly.

10.7.2 Sphenoid stage

The sphenoid ostia are enlarged medially and inferiorly and a "V"-shaped, wide anterior sphenoidotomy is performed [45, 46] The vomer remnant is drilled and the rostrum of the sphenoid sinus is removed [45].

Sphenoidotomy extends from the superior limit of the sphenoid siuns ostium (SO) superiorly to the pterygo-sphenoid synchondrosis/vidian canal at 5 and 7 O'Clock position. By drilling the sphenoid face with these landmarks, the planum sphenoidale, the optico-carotid recess, and the optic protuberances are all well visualized. Laterally it extends to the crest marking the junction of the sphenoid and ethmoid sinuses. A space below the sellar floor should be created to allow free manipulation [45, 46]. Some times it is necessary to extend drilling inferiorly at 6 O'Clock down to clival septum.

The operative space can be further widened by performing posterior ethmoidectomy, this space accommodates the scope, which is named as the cavity and a half technique [47].

When sphenoidotomy is complete, the remaining segment of the vomer demarcates the midline of sellar floor, and the two bulges of carotids are well identified.

At the end of sphenoidotomy, the midline is identified by visualizing the remaining segment of the rostrum (vomer) inferiorly and the middle of the two carotid bulges. The second surgeon then holds the endoscope and acts as a navigator.

10.7.3 Sellar stage

Throughout this stage hemostasis is very important to have a clear surgical field, to visualize important structures and prevent their injury. Sellar floor is drilled out, and a diamond or coarse diamond burr of 3 or 4 mm is used. Low-speed controlled drilling is performed until the floor is as thin as an eggshell. The thinned sellar floor is then broken with a fine spade dissector or a Kerrison number-1 punch [47]. The authors use mushroom punch when available for this step instead of Kerrison punch.

By pressing the sellar dura gently, an estimate of lateral bone removal can be made. Sellar floor and anterior wall are removed millimeter by millimeter circumferentially till four blue lines are seen, superiorly and inferiorly the inter-cavernous sinuses, and laterally the cavernous sinuses) [47].

Firm tumors with suprasellar extension and a dumbbell configuration require an extended approach; in addition to the previously described sphenoidotomy, the tuberculum sellae, planum sphenoidale, and the medial optico-carotid recess are all removed with or without transdiaphragmatic dura opening [48, 49].

Opening of the dura is done in different ways, the rational is to have good surgical access with preservation of the dura, a vertical linear incision with crossed extensions, a cruciate incision which is the preference of the authors, or two vertical incisions joined by a transverse cut (H shaped).

10.7.3.1 Piecemeal tumor removal

A clear surgical field is crucial to perform safe and effective surgery. This is achieved by good hemostasis and saline irrigation; a clear field will allow good visualization. The endoscope enables an accurate detailed view, with step-by-step dissection, choosing appropriate size and good visualization of the tip of the instrument, avoiding blind dissection and traction, these measures prevent injury of the important

DOI: http://dx.doi.org/10.5772/intechopen.1003030

structures; internal carotid artery, optic chiasm/nerves, suprasellar cistern, cavernous sinus, and normal pituitary gland.

The tumor should first be mobilized free in a piecemeal manner, and then gently grasped without traction in a holding forceps of appropriate size. Starting with the basal and posterior part of the tumor, it is removed in a posterior trajectory toward the clivus-dorsum sellae junction in a caudal to rostral direction [41, 45].

Next the lateral portion of the tumor is removed with the upward-angled curettes, lateral curettes are preferred to be used by the authors in clockwise and anticlockwise directions, and a plane of dissection is then created. Lastly, the superior portion of the tumor is removed after making an upward dura cut if required. Tumor decompression is done with a bimanual dissection-curette in the right hand and the suction in the left as in **Figure 13**; or utilizing the double suction method, where the left suction retracts the dura up, and the right suction sucks the tumor [46]. This results in progressive descent of the suprasellar tumor, which is then continuously removed concentrically. The normal pituitary gland is identified as a thinned-out, pinkish, firm tissue plastered to the diaphragma sella and is preserved. While approaching the cavernous sinus medial wall extension of the tumor, the space between the posterior clinoid and the carotid siphon (the reverse S contour) represents an ideal entry point for the removal of tumor from the posterior segment of the cavernous sinus [46]. Bleeding from the cavernous sinuses is controlled with surgical and or gelfoam.

Identification of internal carotids, optic chiasm, and normal pituitary is the safest way to prevent accidental injury. Suprasellar cistern injury infrequently happens leading to CSF leak, this should be detected intraoperatively to reconstruct appropriately.

10.7.3.2 Visualization

At the end of tumor dissection, visualization of tumor bed is very important in searching for a possible residue, an angled endoscope is used, 30 degrees or 45 degrees.

The diaphragma sellae is pushed upwards by cotton patties to expose hidden areas, if the residual tumor is seen, it is dissected from the recess using a curved suction/

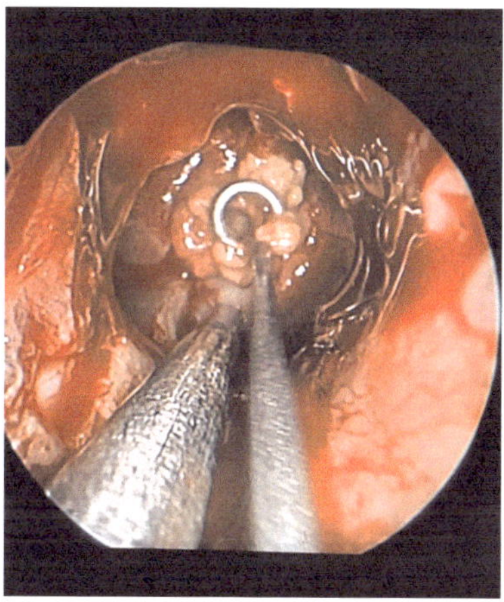

Figure 13.
Trans nasal endoscopic pituitary surgery: Endoscopic view at the stage of tumor dissection, note the curette and suction, three hands technique.

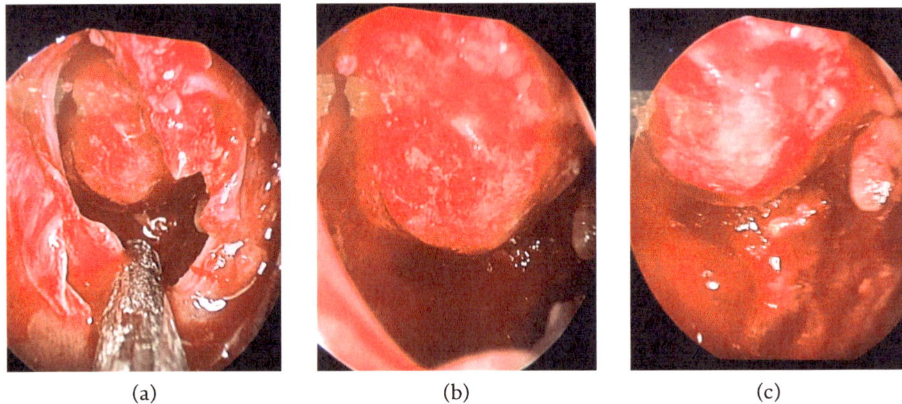

Figure 14.
(a-c) trans nasal endoscopic pituitary surgery: Endoscopic view at the stage of tumor removal. In a zero degree endoscope is used and in b & c 30 ° endoscope is used, note remnant of the tumor at the carotid-optic recess at 3 O'clock.

curette [41, 45]. The angled endoscope is positioned at 6 O'Clock, while the instruments are passed above the endoscope.

The technique is by advancing the angled endoscope close to the target, for accurate visualization, then withdrawing the endoscope while advancing the dissecting instrument gently under vision in a harmonic dynamic fashion [16, 17].

Lastly, the sella is inspected (360 degrees) in a clockwise fashion, starting at 6 O'Clock, and the cavernous sinuses are inspected during endoscope rotation. **Figure 14(A–C)**.

The fact that only 10% of remnant of normal pituitary gland is enough for normal function, makes preservation of the gland a relatively easy step, it appears as a pinkish tissue that is more adherent than adenoma tissue, the site of which is anticipated according to MRI study preoperatively [41, 46].

Finally, the last remaining piece of the tumor is usually located at the insertion of the pituitary stalk [3].

The most common sites that accommodate the residual tumor are under the upper anterior lip of the dura at the level of the anterior cavernous sinus and the angle between optic nerve and carotid artery at the medial optico-carotid recesses [41, 46].

10.7.3.3 Reconstruction stage

The rationale beyond reconstruction is to make a watertight seal that prevents cerebrospinal fluid (CSF) leak, ascending infection, and pneumocephalus. This is achieved by a multilayered repair with fat, fascia or septal cartilage, tissue glue or histocryl, and nasoseptal flap.

Haddad and Bassagasteguy's described the nasoseptal flap in 2006, this flap was a landmark in anterior skull base reconstruction as it is regarded as the workhorse for reconstruction in this region. This flap is the most versatile for reconstruction as it reduces morbidity significantly [50]. The greatest advantage of the nasoseptal flap is the reduction of CSF leak rate. At the beginning of endoscopic endonasal approach, before the advent of the nasoseptal flap, CSF leak rate was 24%, however, CSF leak was much reduced to 3% when nasoseptal flap was utilized in reconstruction according to recent studies [51]. Description of anatomy of the nasoseptal flap, harvesting, and its blood supply is described earlier in this chapter within the nasal stage.

10.7.3.4 Reconstruction steps

Valsava maneuver is performed after tumor resection to check for CSF leak [35, 45]. The first step in reconstruction is filling the tumor cavity with abdominal fat routinely, this prevents CSF leak from delayed rupture of the arachnoid and prevents empty sella syndrome [35].

In case of cerebrospinal fluid leak, the sella may be repaired by fat graft, and making sure that the fat graft is pulsating. An overzealous sellar packing should be avoided [41].

At the level of the dura and deep to osteal defect, a piece of surgicel or facia lata is placed to seal dural incision, in few cases operated on by the authors, a piece of fashioned septal cartilage is placed to tuck in under bony edges, in one case it acted as a trapdoor leading to pneumocephalus, so cartilage when used should be carefully positioned. On top of that plane, tissue glue or histocryl is applied, if hisocryl is used, a piece of surgicel is placed. The last layer of reconstruction is the nasoseptal flap, it is delivered from the nasopharynx, where it had been stored, and extended to cover generously the skull base. If histocryl is used before applying the nasoseptal flap as shown in **Figure 15**, they should be separated by surgical or thinned gelfoam, because necrosis of nasoseptal flap will happen if it is in direct contact with the histocryl.

Mechanical support of nasoseptal flap is achieved by application of gelfoam on top of it, as gelfoam swells, it gently pushes the nasoseptal flap in place. Middle turbinates are then medialized to maintain patency of osteomeatal complex and hence sinus drainage. Nasal packs are optional, it is the authors' routine to apply bilaterally ventilated nasal packs.

11. Emergence from anesthesia

At the end of surgery, the following procedures are performed, removal of pharyngeal packs, suction of oral cavity, extubation of endotracheal tube after regaining

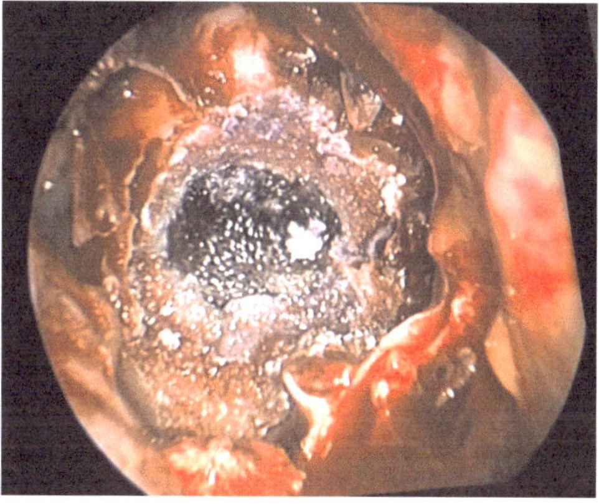

Figure 15.
Trans nasal endoscopic pituitary surgery: Endoscopic view at the stage of reconstruction, note solidification of histocryl at the level of osteal defect at sellar floor.

spontaneous breathing and reflexes. The patient's hemodynamic state should be stabilized. Coughing and straining should be kept to minimum, as both can cause CSF leak, hemorrhage, and dislodgement of nasal packs [28].

11.1 Immediate postoperative care

Care at the end of surgery includes airway management, adequate analgesia, fluid balance control, and endocrine and neurological assessment. Diabetes insipidus and pan hypopituitarism are commonly encountered. Deficiencies in any pituitary hormone must be adequately replaced besides glucocorticoids, this most frequently involves thyroid hormone. Any neurological signs, for example, cranial nerve palsy or visual change should be diagnosed early with further evaluation by imaging or re-exploration.

Diabetes insipidus (DI) if developed, occurs within the first 24 hours postoperatively, this happens when more than 80% of neurons producing vasopressin are destroyed or functionally impaired. Nearly 25% of patients develop transient diabetes insipidus lasting for several days to weeks. In about 0.5% of patients, diabetes insipidus remains permanent [28, 52, 53].

All patients require long-term follow-up with an endocrinologist to assess their hormonal status.

12. Complications

Although transnasal endoscopic pituitary surgery is relatively safe, complications that may develop are serious and some are life-threatening. The complications are related to the preoperative state of the patient e.g., comorbidity and intraoperative events, they are major and minor, acute or long-term.

Immediate post-operative complications are diabetes insipidus (DI), CSF leak, and epistaxis, in that order of frequency, less frequent are endocrine, infection, cardiovascular, and pulmonary. Renal failure and shock are rare, reported complications [54]. Panhypopituitarism and nasal dryness are long-term complications. Management of complications is by a team of endocrine, anesthesia/ICU, and surgery, some complications require urgent surgical intervention e.g. signs of intracranial hemorrhage, vision deterioration, or intractable epistaxis.

12.1 Epistaxis

Epistaxis, when intractable in the immediate postoperative period, requires a return to the operating room to manage rapid loss, control bleeding by electrocautery, and verify the possibility of intracranial hemorrhage, in the latter event revision of surgery is mandatory.

In a series of 557 endoscopic pituitary surgery, posterior nasal septal artery (NSA) was the most common bleeding source of severe postoperative epistaxis following endoscopic transnasal pituitary surgery. To prevent injury of NSA, incision of the septal mucosa should not be extended downward excessively [55]. lowering of sphenoid rostrum should not exceed 5 mm below the lower lip of natural sphenoid sinus ostium, and intraoperative hemostasis should be ensured by bipolar electrocoagulation.

Minor epistaxis from nasal mucosa cut edges, or when unidentified is usually managed by anterior nasal packing, other measures are; the use of intranasal hemostatic agents, or office cauterization in delayed epistaxis that can happen up to 3 weeks postoperatively [56].

12.2 CSF leak

The incidence of postoperative CSF Leak after endoscopic treatment of pituitary adenoma is between 0.5% and 14% [57, 58]. The risk of developing CSF leak is associated with intrinsic patient factors with statistical significance, these are: age more than 65 years, male, body mass index more than 25, and multiple comorbidities. The prevalence of CSF leaks was not associated with expertise availability, hospital stay, volume of operations in the institute, and teaching status: whether it is a teaching hospital or not [59, 60].

Treatment of CSF leak: For the management of CSF rhinorrhoea after transsphenoidal surgery, procedures using fibrin glue, gelatin gelfoam, and autologous fat graft are effective [61].

Conservative measures by reducing straining and coughing are important. Controversy exists regarding lumbar puncture in management of CSF leak, as an adjunct to surgical repair; it is not favorable by the authors as it carries a risk of meningitis. Prevention of CSF leaks is by identification of leaks intraoperatively and sellar floor reconstruction [62].

12.3 Diabetes insipidus

Diabetes insipidus (DI) is a common complication after transnasal endoscopic pituitary surgery. It has been reported that the incidence of DI after TEPS is 0.9%–36.1% [63]. During tumor resection, injury of the neurons that produce and transport vasopressin (magnocellular neurons) lead to DI, these neurons form the hypothalamo-hypophyseal tract leading to a transient or permanent imbalance in water homeostasis [64].

Nayak et al. [65] found that tumor size, suprasellar extension, and preoperative visual abnormalities are significantly correlated with the postoperative DI ($P < 0.05$). In addition, Winzeler et al. [66] confirmed that a low serum peptide level at 12 hours after surgery is a strong predictor of DI.

Transient DI typically occurs within 24–48 hours after the operation and usually remits spontaneously within 3–5 days [67, 68].

Patients are diagnosed with DI and treated with desmopressin (1-diamino-8-arginine vasopressin) when urine output is less than 5 mL/kg/hr. With a serum sodium concentration of more than 145 mmol/L or an increase of more than 3 mmol/L in serum sodium concentration between two consecutive tests after surgery. DI is considered permanent if medical treatment is required for more than 6 months after surgery [66].

13. Current study

13.1 Objectives

A pilot study was conducted to investigate the demographic data, clinical presentation, surgical management, and complications of pituitary tumors in a single center in Khartoum.

13.2 Methodology

This is a retrospective, analytic, hospital-based study. Conducted in Ribat University Hospital, Neuro Spine Center, Khartoum, Sudan. From November 2017 to March 2023.

Study subjects: Patients presented to the outpatient department with symptoms and signs of sellar pathology and upon radiological assessment have evidence of pituitary tumor, or patients referred from: ophthalmology department with vision affection, endocrine department with abnormal hormone profile, or obstetrics and gynecology department with infertility. A multidisciplinary team evaluated the patients by clinical, radiological, laboratory and detailed ophthalmological assessment, the team consists of members from the following departments: neurosurgery, ophthalmology, endocrinology, otolaryngology, radiology, anesthesiology, and ICU. Oncology and Obstetrics and gynecology were often required. The plan of management was then set for each patient, including a lifelong follow up plan.

Inclusion criteria: Patients with pituitary tumors that were proven radiologically and performed assessment by the multidisciplinary team. Patients who underwent transnasal endoscopic pituitary surgery according to the decision of the team, with the indications mentioned in this text.

Exclusion criteria: patients with sellar lesions other than pituitary tumors, e.g., chordoma, craniopharyngioma, meningioma ... etc. and patients planned for external (craniotomy) approach.

A data sheet was used to collect the information.

Surgical procedure: A transnasal endoscopic pituitary surgery was performed according to the described technique and details mentioned in the surgical section earlier.

13.3 Results

A total of 162 patients were included in this study, 150 were pituitary adenoma, and 12 patients were other pathologies: three meningioma, one retroclival epidrmoid cyst, 6 craniopharyngioma, one arachnoid cyst, and one fungal granuloma.

The ages ranged between 19 and 76 years. Males and females were almost equal. Regarding the clinical presentation, vision impairment was the leading, it was reported in 137 patients (91%), 6 patients (4%) presented with acromegaly, due to excessive growth hormone production, and 7 patients (4.6%) with hyperprolactinemia. Three patients (2%) presented with apoplexy. Tumor extension according to MRI: 25 (17%) tumors were confined to the sella and 125 (83%) tumors extended to supra and/or parasellar regions. During the COVID-19 pandemic, as recommended by most of the guidelines to cease elective surgeries, only two emergency patients were operated on, one presented with apoplexy, was a young general surgeon, presented with severe headache and acute failing vision for 2 days, surgery was performed after 24 hours only of presentation, his vision was saved immediately postoperatively and his career so. The second emergency patient presented with hydrocephalus, he required external ventricular drainage before endoscopic transnasal surgery.

The operative time at the beginning was an average of 6 hours, it decreased to 2.5 hours after 3 years from the beginning, however, surgery was lengthened in tumors with suprasellar and parasellar extension even lately.

Complications were: diabetes insipidus in 6 patients (4%), in five of them DI was transient, CSF leak that required re-exploration and reconstruction was reported in 3

DOI: http://dx.doi.org/10.5772/intechopen.1003030

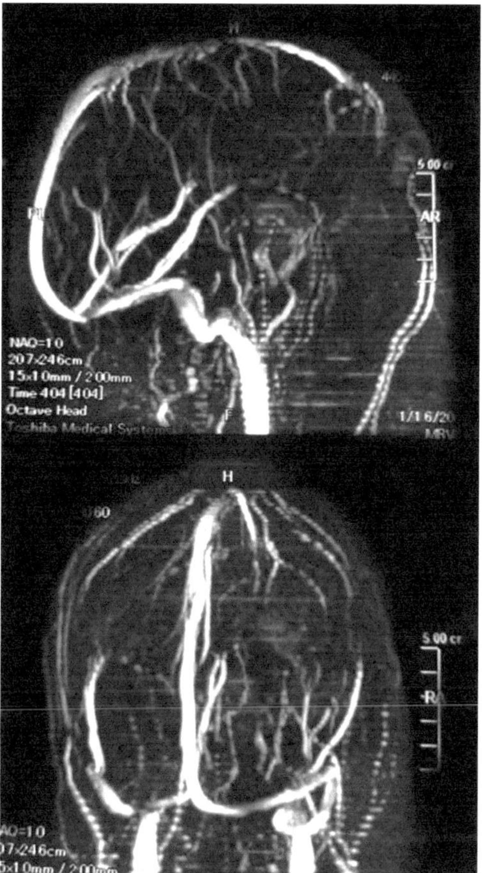

Figure 16.
MR Venography, demonstrating superior sagittal sinus thrombosis.

patients (2%), tension pneumocephalus and CSF leak in one patient (0.7%), chest infection in one patient, superior sagittal sinus thrombosis in one patient as shown in **Figure 16**. Visual symptoms improved in 128 patients (93%), and the remaining 9 patients who showed no improvement in vision, their vision were affected for more than 6 months when surgery was performed. Panhypopituitarism was reported in one patient. The mortality rate is 2% (3 patients), one intraoperative death due to massive uncontrolled bleeding (25 years male), one DI and one died of aspiration pneumonia postoperatively.

Three patients required revision surgery for tumor recurrence. One patient required a planned external approach after endoscopic transnasal resection, while two patients had symptomatic and radiological tumor recurrence. No reported vision deterioration, persistent anosmia, or internal carotid injury.

Gross tumor resection and outcome of surgery are still under prospective study and will be reported somewhere else.

13.4 Discussion

In the current study, a variety of lesions were encountered in the sellar region, reflecting the variety of anatomical structures at histological level, and diversity of embryological origin, apart from pituitary adenoma, lesions included meningioma, chordoma, craniopharyngioma. One case was found to be fungal granuloma which extended from the sphenoid sinus, mimicking pituitary adenoma, an important differential diagnosis. Lesions of the sellar region present as early as childhood, for example, craniopharyngioma, it is not uncommon, where six cases of craniopharyngioma were diagnosed among the studied patients. Radiological findings are a very important tool for making preoperative diagnosis of lesions other than pituitary adenoma, a neuroradiologist is an important team member, where expertise and opinion are very crucial in preoperative diagnosis, and hence management plan, a combined multidisciplinary discussion, at the time of deciding the plan of management has great input.

In low-resource countries where there is paucity of medical services, as the authors experience, most of the patients are referred from ophthalmology departments with visual complications, where adenoma is huge in size, **Figure 3**, demonstrates adenoma on MRI pushing the optic chiasm.

The majority present with large or giant tumors upon radiological assessment with suprasellar and parasellar extensions.

One patient presented with hydrocephalus because the tumor was enormous to the extent that it extended superiorly leading to obstruction of the third ventricle as the patient was initially managed by external ventricular drainage, and then scheduled for elective endoscopic pituitary resection. This patient reflects the advanced clinical manifestations of pituitary adenoma in the studied series.

Elective endoscopic transnasal surgeries were recommended to be paused during the COVID 19 era [69], during that period elective transnasal endoscopic pituitary surgeries were postponed.

One of the three apoplexy patients was a doctor, he presented with severe headache for 2 days, and had deterioration in vision for 1 day, otherwise, he was dealing a normal life, with no significant medical history, upon MRI brain, pituitary macroadenoma was detected, within the next 24 hours of presentation, he was thoroughly investigated, where it was a nonfunctioning adenoma, vision impairment started the second day of headache, this signifies that hemorrhage was progressive and hematoma was rapidly increasing in size, he was operated on within 24 hours, and showed immediate improvement in vision and headache in the postoperative period. This case is another example of an emergency pituitary surgery.

The learning curve of endoscopic transnasal pituitary surgery was obvious and well demonstrated by the reduction of operative time to almost one-third. This is achieved by the acquisition of surgical skills, catching surgical tips and tricks, and forming harmony between operating team members. With experience more complicated cases are operated on, these include parasellar and suprasellar tumors, meticulous dissection of these tumors requires a longer duration, to avoid injury of the neighboring structures, namely the carotids, optic chiasm, optic nerve, cavernous sinus, cistern, and normal pituitary gland, special technique is advocated and described earlier in the surgical section. Utilization of angled endoscopes improves surgical field exposure and is anticipated to minimize the frequency of residual tumors.

The safest and cheapest way to avoid complications is by adequate knowledge of the detailed anatomy, anatomical variations, and surgical landmarks. Image guidance (neuro-navigation) is used to identify the bony landmarks, it is important especially when anatomical variations are present, nevertheless, it is not a substitute for knowledge, it is rather an adjunct, that helps increase safety and reduce operative time.

Because our hospital is a limited facility, neuro-navigation is not provided routinely, we depend mainly on knowledge of anatomy and surgical skills.

In this study, four patients out of 150 cases required surgical intervention, with a rate of CSF leak of 2.7% only, this low rate is most likely due to the reconstruction multilayer protocol which is described earlier; two important layers are abdominal fat and nasoseptal flap, both are used routinely in reconstruction during primary surgery.

One patient developed CSF leak and deterioration in the level of consciousness after a smooth and full recovery from anesthesia, 12 hours postoperatively, on MRI, tension pneumocephalus was demonstrated. Generally in reconstruction as mentioned earlier, multilayers are used, at the level of the osteal defect of the sellar floor, fashioned septal cartilage is used, and tucked in beneath the bony edges of the sella, in this particular patient the cartilage acted as a trapdoor allowing the escape of CSF and permitting air to enter simultaneously, this patient required emergency revision and reconstruction, he improved clinically and radiologically and was discharged from the ICU 3 days later. This case is a good example of the importance of early emergence from anesthesia, where neurological signs are indicative of intracranial complications. Panhypopituitarism was reported in one patient, but due to missing data, as this is a pilot study, a future prospective study, is expected to report hypopituitarism among patients more frequently.

One patient developed superior sagittal thrombosis in the postoperative period. This complication was reported in a revision case with endoscopic transnasal surgery [70].

14. Conclusion

Pituitary tumors present with ophthalmic and compression effects, these include vision impairment and hydrocephalus, while nonfunctioning adenoma present with excess hormone production, other sellar pathologies are frequently encountered, these include meningioma, craniopharyngioma, and arachnoid cyst. Pituitary tumors occur in a wide age range, Acute hemorrhage in pituitary adenoma presents with severe headache and acute failing vision, in the current study it was reported in 2% of patients. Radiological investigations are important for preoperative diagnosis and planning and image-guided monitoring is advocated as routine or at least for patients with unfavorable anatomical variations.

Endoscopic transnasal pituitary surgery nowadays is the gold standard surgery for most pituitary tumors even those with sellar and suprasellar extension, the endoscope has greatly revolutionized pituitary surgery, being minimally invasive and giving superlative visualization of the surgical field when compared to the microscope, especially the corners, furthermore, angled endoscopes display hidden recesses at the tumor site clearly. On the other hand, the learning curve of endoscopic transnasal approach is a steep curve. With experience, the operative time is reduced, surgical outcome is improved, complications are decreased, and more extensive pathology is dealt with. Perioperative management requires a team approach from different specialties related to pituitary pathology. Indications of urgent surgery are apoplexy and hydrocephalus.

Complications of transnasal endoscopic surgery encountered in this study are CSF leak, diabetes insipidus, pneumocephalus, aspiration pneumonia, superior sagittal thrombosis, and death. Vision improvement is not expected when surgery is delayed. Gross tumor resection and revision surgery need to be verified with a detailed longitudinal study.

Author details

Nazik Abdullah[1,2*], Haytham Osman[3,4*], Honida Ibrahim[3*], Khalid Elzein[4,5] and Ali Awad[3]

1 Khartoum ENT Hospital, Khartoum, Sudan

2 Department of Otolaryngology, University of Khartoum, Khartoum, Sudan

3 Ribat University Hospital, Neurosurgery Center, Khartoum, Sudan

4 Department of Surgery, The National Ribat University, Khartoum, Sudan

5 Otolaryngology Department, Ribat University Hospital, Khartoum, Sudan

*Address all correspondence to: nazikfad1223@yahoo.co.uk; haytham2ta@hotmail.com and honida2075@gmail.com

IntechOpen

References

[1] Ganapathy MK, Tadi P. Anatomy, Head and Neck, Pituitary Gland. Treasure Island (FL): StatPearls Publishing; 2023. Available from: https://www.ncbi.nlm.nih.gov/books/nbk551529/

[2] Chin BM, Orlandi RR, Wiggins RH. Evaluation of the sellar and parasellar regions. Magnetic Resonance Imaging Clinics of North America. 2012;**20**(3): 515-543

[3] Larkin S, Ansorge O. Development and Microscopic Anatomy of the Pituitary Gland. In: Feingold KR, Anawalt B, Blackman MR, et al., editors. MDText.com, Inc., South Dartmouth (MA): 2017

[4] Yamashita S, Resende LA, Trindade AP, Zanini MA. A radiologic morphometric study of sellar, infrassellar and parasellar regions by magnetic resonance in adults. Springerplus. 2014;**3**:291

[5] Ceylan S, Anik I, Koc K, Kokturk S, Ceylan S, Cine N, et al. Microsurgical anatomy of membranous layers of the pituitary gland and the expression of extracellular matrix collagenous proteins. Acta Neurochirurgica. 2011;**153**(12):2435-2443 discussion 2443

[6] Ilahi S, Ilahi TB. Anatomy, Adenohypophysis (Pars Anterior, Anterior Pituitary). Treasure Island (FL): StatPearls Publishing; 2022

[7] Go JL, Rajamohan AG. Imaging of the sella and parasellar region. Radiologic Clinics of North America. 2017;**55**(1): 83-101

[8] Lechan RM, Toni R. Functional Anatomy of the Hypothalamus and Pituitary. In: Feingold KR, Anawalt B, Blackman MR, et al., editors. Mdtext.com, Inc.; South Dartmouth (MA): 2016

[9] El Sayed SA, Fahmy MW, Schwartz J. Physiology, Pituitary Gland. Treasure Island (FL): StatPearls Publishing; 2023

[10] Ooi GT, Tawadros N, Escalona RM. Pituitary cell lines and their endocrine applications. Molecular and Cellular Endocrinology. 2004;**228**(1–2):1-21

[11] Fujimoto M, Takeuchi K, Sugimoto M, Maruo T. Prevention of postpartum hemorrhage by uterotonic agents: Comparison of oxytocin and methylergometrine in the management of the third stage of labor. Acta Obstetricia et Gynecologica Scandinavica. 2006;**85**(11):1310-1314

[12] Jost A, Das MJ. Neuroanatomy, Pars Nervosa. Treasure Island (FL): StatPearls Publishing; 2022

[13] Perez-Castro C, Renner U, Haedo MR, Stalla GK, Arzt E. Cellular and molecular specificity of pituitary gland physiology. Physiological Reviews. 2012;**92**(1):1-38

[14] Zada G, Woodmansee WW, Ramkissoon S, Amadio J, Nose V, Laws ER Jr. Atypical pituitary adenomas: Incidence, clinical characteristics, and implications. Journal of Neurosurgery. 2011;**114**:336-344

[15] Al-Shraim M, Asa SL. The 2004 World Health Organization classification of pituitary tumors: What is new? Acta Neuropathologica. 2006;**111**:1-7

[16] Theodros D, Patel M, Ruzevick J, Lim M, Bettegowda C. Pituitary

adenomas: Historical perspective, surgical management and future directions. CNS Oncology. 2015;**4**(06): 411-429

[17] Hardy J. Transphenoidal microsurgery of the normal and pathological pituitary. Clinical Neurosurgery. 1969;**16**:185-217

[18] Molitch ME. Diagnosis and treatment of pituitary adenomas: A review. Journal of the American Medical Association. 2017;**317**(5): 516-524

[19] Freda PU, Beckers AM, Katznelson L, Molitch ME, Montori VM, Post KD, et al. Pituitary incidentaloma: An endocrine society clinical practice guideline. The Journal of Clinical Endocrinology and Metabolism. 2011; **96**(4):894-904

[20] Ferrante E, Ferraroni M, Castrignanò T, Menicatti L, Anagni M, Reimondo G, et al. Non-functioning pituitary adenoma database: A useful resource to improve the clinical management of pituitary tumors. European Journal of Endocrinology. 2006;**155**(6):823-829

[21] Ogra S, Nichols AD, Stylli S, Kaye AH, Savino PJ, Danesh-Meyer HV. Visual acuity and pattern of visual field loss at presentation in pituitary adenoma. Journal of Clinical Neuroscience. 2014;**21**(5): 735-740

[22] Steiner E, Wimberger D, Imhof H, Knosp E, Hajek P. Gd-DTPA in the MR diagnosis of pituitary adenomas. Rofo. 1989;**150**(3):323-327

[23] Kucharczyk W, Bishop JE, Plewes DB, Keller MA, George S. Detection of pituitary microadenomas: Comparison of dynamic keyhole fast spin-echo, unenhanced, and conventional contrast-enhanced MR imaging. AJR. American Journal of Roentgenology. 1994;**163**(3): 671-679

[24] Evanson J. In: Feingold KR, Anawalt B, Blackman MR, et al., editors. Radiology of the Pituitary. South Dartmouth (MA): Mdtext.com, Inc.; 2000. Available from: https://www.ncbi.nlm.nih.gov/books/nbk279161/

[25] Russ S, Anastasopoulou C, Shafiq I. Pituitary Adenoma. Treasure Island (FL): StatPearls Publishing; 2023. Available from: https://www.ncbi.nlm.nih.gov/books/nbk554451/

[26] Bhimani AD, Schupper AJ, Arnone GD, Chada D, Chaker AN, Mohammadi N, et al. Size matters: Rethinking of the sizing classification of pituitary adenomas based on the rates of surgery: A multi-institutional retrospective study of 29,651 patients. Journal of Neurological Surgery Part B: Skull Base. 2020;**83**(1):66-75. DOI: 10.1055/s-0040-1716673

[27] Horvat A, Kolak J, Gopčević A, Ilej M, Gnjidić Ž. Anesthetic management of patients undergoing pituitary surgery. Acta Clinica Croatica. 2011;**50**:209-216

[28] Burton CM, Nemergut EC. Anesthetic and critical care management of patients undergoing pituitary surgery. Frontiers of Hormone Research. 2006; **34**:236-255

[29] Duz B, Harman F, Secer HI, Bolu E, Gonul E. Transsphenoidal approaches to the pituitary: A progression in experience in a single centre. Acta Neurochirurgica. 2008;**150**:1133-1138

[30] Jagannthan J, Laws ER, Jane JA Jr. Advantages of endoscopic approach and

transitioning from microscope to the endoscope for endonasal approaches. In: Kassam AB, Gardner PA, editors. Endoscopic Approaches for Skull Base. Basel, Switzerland: S. Karger AG; 2012. pp. 7-20

[31] Musleh W, Sonabend AM, Lesniak MS. Role of craniotomy in the management of pituitary adenomas and sellar/parasellar tumors. Expert Review of Anticancer Therapy. 2006;**6**(Suppl 9): S79-S83. DOI: 10.1586/14737140.6.9s.S79

[32] Salama MM, Rady MR. Transcranial approaches for pituitary adenomas: Current indications and clinical and radiological outcomes. Egyptian Journal of Neurosurgery. 2021;**36**:21. DOI: 10.1186/s41984-021-00117-x

[33] Ojha BK, Husain M, Rastogi M, Chandra A, Chugh A, Husain N. Combined trans-sphenoidal and simultaneous trans-ventricular-endoscopic decompression of a giant pituitary adenoma: Case report. Acta Neurochirurgica. 2009;**151**(7):843-847; discussion 847. DOI: 10.1007/s00701-009-0336-z Epub 2009 Apr 28

[34] Leach P, Abou-Zeid AH, Kearney T, Davis J, Trainer PJ, Gnanalingham KK. Endoscopic transsphenoidal pituitary surgery: Evidence of an operative learning curve. Neurosurgery. 2010;**67**: 1205-1212

[35] O'Malley BW Jr, Grady MS, Gabel BC, Cohen MA, Heuer GG, Pisapia J, et al. Comparison of endoscopic and microscopic removal of pituitary adenomas: Single-surgeon experience and the learning curve. Neurosurgical Focus. 2008;**25**:E10

[36] Huang J, Hong X, Cai Z, Lv Q, Jiang Y, Dai W, et al. The learning curve of endoscopic endonasal transsphenoidal surgery for pituitary adenomas with different surgical complexity. Frontiers in Surgery. 2023;**10**:1117766. DOI: 10.3389/fsurg.2023.1117766

[37] Okuda T, Kataoka K, Kato A. Training in endoscopic endonasal transsphenoidal surgery using a skull model and eggs. Acta Neurochirurgica. 2010;**152**:1801-1804

[38] Sharma BS, Sawarkar DP, Suri A. Endoscopic pituitary surgery: Techniques, tips and tricks, nuances, and complication avoidance. Neurology India. 2016;**64**:724-736

[39] Cappabianca P, Cavallo LM, de Divitiis E. Endoscopic endonasal transsphenoidal surgery. Neurosurgery. 2004;**55**:933-940

[40] Cavallo LM, Dal Fabbro M, Jalalod'din H, Messina A, Esposito I, Esposito F, et al. Endoscopic endonasal transsphenoidal surgery. Before scrubbing in: Tips and tricks. Surgical Neurology. 2007;**67**:342-347

[41] Ezzat S, Asa SL, Couldwell WT, Barr CE, Dodge WE, Vance ML, et al. The prevalence of pituitary adenomas: A systematic review. Cancer. 2004;**101**: 613-619

[42] Laws ER Jr, Lopes MB. The new WHO classification of pituitary tumors: Highlights and areas of controversy. Acta Neuropathologica. 2006;**111**:80-81

[43] Jho HD, Alfieri A. Endoscopic endonasal pituitary surgery: Evolution of surgical technique and equipment in 150 operations. Minimally Invasive Neurosurgery. 2001;**44**:1-12

[44] Sigler AC, D'Anza B, Lobo BC, Woodard TD, Recinos PF, Sindwani R. Endoscopic skull base reconstruction: An evolution of materials and methods.

Otolaryngologic Clinics of North America. 2017;**50**(3):643-653

[45] Reuter G, Bouchain O, Demanez L, Scholtes F, Martin D. Skull base reconstruction with pedicled nasoseptal flap: Technique, indications, and limitations. Journal of Cranio-Maxillo-Facial Surgery. 2019;**47**(1):29-32

[46] Lucas JW, Zada G. Endoscopic surgery for pituitary tumors. Neurosurgery Clinics of North America. 2012;**23**:555-569

[47] Kassam A, Snyderman CH, Mintz A, Gardner P, Carrau RL. Expanded endonasal approach: The rostrocaudal axis. Part I. Crista galli to the sella turcica. Neurosurgical Focus. 2005;**19**:E3

[48] Kassam AB, Gardner PA, Prevedello DM, Snyderman CH, Carrau RL, Zhao B. Principles of endoneurosurgery. In: Kassam AB, Gardner PA, editors. Endoscopic Approaches for Skull Base. Basel, Switzerland: S. Karger AG; 2012. pp. 21-26

[49] Sankhla SK, Jayashankar N, Khan GM. Surgical management of selected pituitary macroadenomas using extended endoscopic endonasal transsphenoidal approach: Early experience. Neurology India. 2013;**61**: 122-130

[50] Zhao B, Wei YK, Li GL, Li YN, Yao Y, Kang J, et al. Extended transsphenoidal approach for pituitary adenomas invading the anterior cranial base, cavernous sinus, and clivus: A single-center experience with 126 consecutive cases. Journal of Neurosurgery. 2010;**112**:108-117

[51] Zanation AM, Carrau RL, Snyderman CH, Germanwala AV, Gardner PA, Prevedello DM, et al. Nasoseptal flap reconstruction of high flow intraoperative cerebral spinal fluid leaks during endoscopic skull base surgery. American Journal of Rhinology & Allergy. 2009;**23**(5):518-521

[52] Singh C, Shah N. Posterior nasoseptal flap in the reconstruction of skull base defects following endonasal surgery. The Journal of Laryngology and Otology. 2019;**133**(5):380-385

[53] Nemergut EC, Dumont AS, Barry UT, Laws ER. Perioperative management of patients undergoing transsphenoidal pituitary surgery. Anesthesia and Analgesia. 2005;**101**: 1170-1181

[54] Gnjidi ć Ž. Suvremeno kirurško liječenje tumora selarne regije. Liječnički Vjesnik. 2004;**126**:26-31

[55] Al-Qurayshi Z, Bennion DM, Greenlee JDW, Graham SM. Endoscopic pituitary surgery: National database review. Head & Neck. 2022;**44**(12): 2678-2685

[56] Liu X, Wang P, Li M, Chen G. Incidence, risk factors, management and prevention of severe postoperative epistaxis after endoscopic endonasal transsphenoidal surgery: A single center experience. Frontiers in Surgery. 2023; **10**:1203409. DOI: 10.3389/fsurg.2023.1203409

[57] Zimmer LA, Andaluz N. Incidence of epistaxis after endoscopic pituitary surgery: Proposed treatment algorithm. Ear, Nose, & Throat Journal. 2018;**97**(3): E44-E48

[58] Rotman LE, Alford EN, Davis MC, Vaughan TB, Woodworth BA, Riley KO. Preoperative radiographic and clinical factors associated with the visualization of intraoperative cerebrospinal fluid

during endoscopic transsphenoidal resection of pituitary adenomas. Surgical Neurology International. 2020;**11**:59

[59] Cohen S, Jones SH, Dhandapani S, Negm HM, Anand VK, Schwartz TH. Lumbar drains decrease the risk of postoperative cerebrospinal fluid leak following endonasal endoscopic surgery for suprasellar meningiomas in patients with high body mass index. Operative Neurosurgery. 2018;**14**(1): 66-71

[60] Zhou Z, Zuo F, Chen X, et al. Risk factors for postoperative cerebrospinal fluid leakage after transsphenoidal surgery for pituitary adenoma: A meta-analysis and systematic review. BMC Neurology. 2021;**21**:417. DOI: 10.1186/s12883-021-02440-0

[61] Zhang C, Ding X, Lu Y, Hu L, Hu G. Cerebrospinal fluid rhinorrhoea following transsphenoidal surgery for pituitary adenoma: Experience in a Chinese centre. Acta Otorhinolaryngologica Italica. 2017; **37**(4):303-307. DOI: 10.14639/0392-100X-1086

[62] Ahn S, Park JS, Kim DH, Kim SW, Jeun SS. Surgical experience in prevention of postoperative CSF leaks using abdominal fat grafts in endoscopic endonasal transsphenoidal surgery for pituitary adenomas. Journal of Neurological Surgery Part B: Skull Base. 2021;**82**(5):522-527. DOI: 10.1055/s-0040-1712179 Epub 2020 Aug 20

[63] Schreckinger M, Szerlip N, Mittal S. Diabetes insipidus following resection of pituitary tumors. Clinical Neurology and Neurosurgery. 2013;**115**(2):121-126. DOI: 10.1016/j.clineuro.2012.08.009 ISSN 0303-8467. Available from: https://www.sciencedirect.com/science/article/pii/s0303846712004349

[64] Christodoulou E, Ma J, Collins GS, Steyerberg EW, Verbakel JY, Van Calster B. A systematic review shows no performance benefit of machine learning over logistic regression for clinical prediction models. Journal of Clinical Epidemiology. 2019;**110**:12-22. DOI: 10.1016/j.jclinepi.2019.02.004 ISSN 0895-4356. Available from: https://www.sciencedirect.com/science/article/pii/s0895435618310813

[65] de Vries F, Lobatto DJ, Verstegen MJT, van Furth WR, Pereira AM, Biermasz NR. Postoperative diabetes insipidus: How to define and grade this complication? Pituitary. 2021; **24**(2):284-291. DOI: 10.1007/s11102-020-01083-7 Epub 2020 Sep 29

[66] Oh H, Cheun H, Kim YJ, Yoon HK, Kang H, Lee HC, et al. Cephalocaudal tumor diameter is a predictor of diabetes insipidus after endoscopic transsphenoidal surgery for non-functioning pituitary adenoma. Pituitary. 2021;**24**(3):303-311. DOI: 10.1007/s11102-020-01108-1 Epub 2020 Nov 16

[67] Zhan R, Ma Z, Wang D, Li X. Pure endoscopic endonasal transsphenoidal approach for nonfunctioning pituitary adenomas in the elderly: Surgical outcomes and complications in 158 patients. World Neurosurgery. 2015; **84**(6):1572-1578, ISSN 1878-8750. DOI: 10.1016/j.wneu.2015.08.035. Available from: https://www.sciencedirect.com/science/article/pii/s1878875015010517

[68] Lobatto DJ, de Vries F, Zamanipoor Najafabadi AH, Pereira AM, Peul WC, Vliet Vlieland TPM, et al. Preoperative risk factors for postoperative complications in endoscopic pituitary surgery: A systematic review. Pituitary. 2018;**21**(1):84-97. DOI: 10.1007/s11102-017-0839-1

[69] Kamel R, Ragab A, Abdelghaffar H, Kaled A, Fattah AEA, Abdelaziz M, et al. Safe practice guidance: A review for otorhinolaryngologists during COVID-19 pandemic and after reopen process. Rhinology Online. 2020;**3**:128-140. DOI: 10.4193/RHINOL/20.014

[70] Thakur JD, Corlin A, Mallari RJ, Yawitz S, Eisenberg A, Sivakumar W, et al. Complication avoidance protocols in endoscopic pituitary adenoma surgery: A retrospective cohort study in 514 patients. Pituitary. 2021;**24**(6): 930-942. DOI: 10.1007/s11102-021-01167-y Epub 2021 Jul 2

Chapter 3

Endoscopic Endonasal Approach for Tuberculum-Planum Sphenoidale Meningioma

Md Al Amin Salek, Rukun Uddin Chowdhury, Ahmed-Ul-Mursalin Chaudhury, Amir Alim, Abdul Hye Manik, Hasnain Faisal, Shamantha Afreen, Nwoshin Jahan and Rajib Sahriar

Abstract

Meningioma is the most common type of primary brain tumor, accounting for approximately 30% of all brain tumors. Anterior skull base meningiomas represent 8.8% of all meningiomas. They can be in olfactory groove, planum sphenoidale, or tuberculum sellae region. Their approach is challenging, tuberculum-planum sphenoidale meningiomas are a subgroup that can be approached and resected by using an endoscopic endonasal corridor. The complex anatomy in relation to important neurovascular structures poses difficulties in the resection of these lesions endonasally. Moreover, surgically created skull base defect closure is crucial for prevention of CSF leaks. In this chapter, the technical nuances and outcome of this approach are described.

Keywords: endoscopic, endonasal, tuberculum-planum sphenoidale, meningioma, outcome

1. Introduction

Anterior skull base meningiomas originate from different locations (olfactory groove [OG], planum sphenoidale [PS], tuberculum sellae [TS], parasellar region, or anterior clinoid. Tuberculum sella and planum sphenoidale meningiomas represent 5–10% of intracranial meningiomas [1]. Its incidence is common in the fourth decade of life. Female is more affected than male by this tumor. Due to their anatomical location, tuberculum sellae meningiomas play a significant role in the compression of the optic pathway. TS meningioma classically presents with "the chiasmal syndrome", a primary optic atrophy with bitemporal field defect due to variable compression on the optic pathway. PS meningiomas are located more anterior and in proximity to the olfactory groove location so visual disturbances are uncommon. The pituitary hormone functions usually remain within normal limits. In neuroimaging the sella remains normal as the tumor 0riginates exclusively from tuberculum sella and planum sphenoidale. Conventionally craniotomy and surgical decompression are the mainstay of treatment [2]. With the advancement of neuroimaging, neuro navigation, and optics, the endoscopic endonasal transsphenoidal approach is a favuorable surgical corridor for tuberculum sella and planum sphenoidale meningioma [3]. Without brain retraction and direct attack to the vascular supply, endoscopic endonasal transsphenoidal resection is a useful surgical option for TS and PS meningioma management as well as visual recovery [4].

In this chapter, the technical pearl and the outcome of endoscopic endonasal transsphenoidal approach for the management of TS and PS meningiomas will be described.

2. Materials and methods

Retrospective analysis of TS and PS meningioma which underwent endoscopic endonasal transsphenoidal approach. The surgical access was through transtubercular-transplanum corridor. In the study, there were a total of 12 cases in a period of 8 years. TS meningiomas were located on the small surface between the chiasmatic sulcus and diaphragm sellae, and PS meningiomas, those located more anteriorly (**Figure 1a** and **b**).

All the patients in the study group had been examined preoperatively with computed tomography (CT) and magnetic resonance imaging (MRI) studies. Ophthalmological and endocrinological evaluations were done in all cases.

The indications for endoscopic approaches were tumors situated on TS-PS region in the midline with or without extension into the optic canal and vessel encasement. Those cases which underwent craniotomy, olfactory groove region tumor, a large tumor extending beyond the mid pupillary line were excluded both preoperatively and postoperatively.

In follow-up protocol clinical, radiological, and ophthalmological outcomes were recorded initially 3 monthly and 6 monthly for 2 years and then every year to rule out any recurrence. The outcomes were analyzed and recorded for each case individually.

3. Surgical steps

Preoperative counseling for the endoscopic endonasal approach was recorded as per standard protocol.

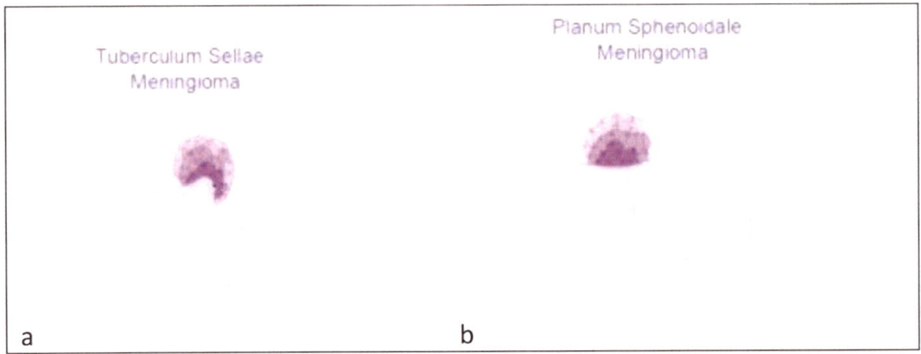

Figure 1.
(a) Tuberculum sella (TS) meningioma and (b) planum sphenoidale (PS) meningioma [5, 6].

Anesthesia: General anesthesia with orotracheal intubation.

Position: Supine position. The head was fixed by Mayfield head clamp and tilted to the left (**Figure 2**).

Preparation of nasal cavity: Normal saline and chlorhexidine gluconate were used for antiseptic wash. For vasoconstriction, adrenalin (1:1000) soaked cottonoids were used for at least 5 min.

Instruments: 4-mm rigid endoscopes with 0°, 30°, and 70° angled lenses.

Steps: The patient together with the endoscopic/video camera equipment is draped with aseptic techniques. Fascia lata and free fat graft were prepared from the thigh. The vascularized nasoseptal flap (Hadad flap) was raised. The surgical corridor was created by doing middle turbinectomy, removal of both the posterior bony septum and anterior cartilaginous septum, shoulder osteotomy, and removal of the vomer. The mucosa of the sphenoid sinus was removed to expose the sellar anatomy. Intra-op vascular Doppler was used to locate the ICA-to-ICA area. An electric drill was used to remove the bony area of TS-PS region and expose the dura over the tumor base.

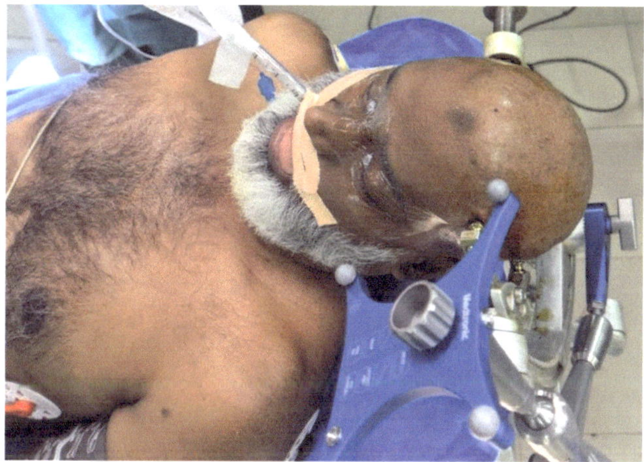

Figure 2.
Position-supine and head were fixed by Mayfield head clamp.

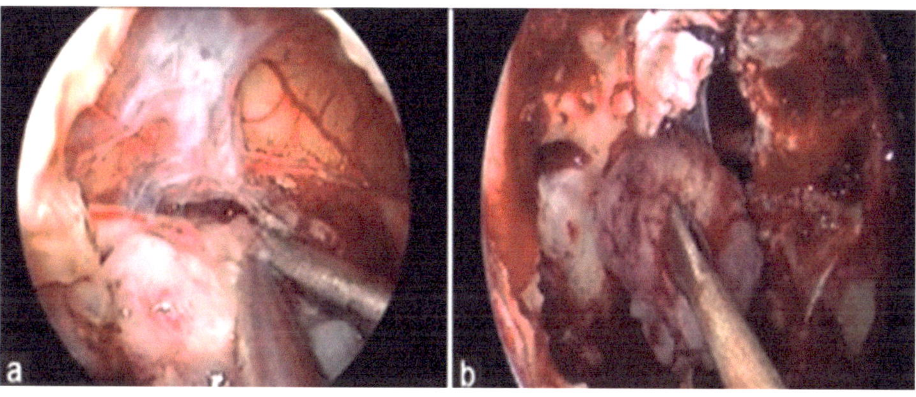

Figure 3.
Intraoperative removal of tumors (a) tumor arachnoid interphase and (b) delivery of tumor.

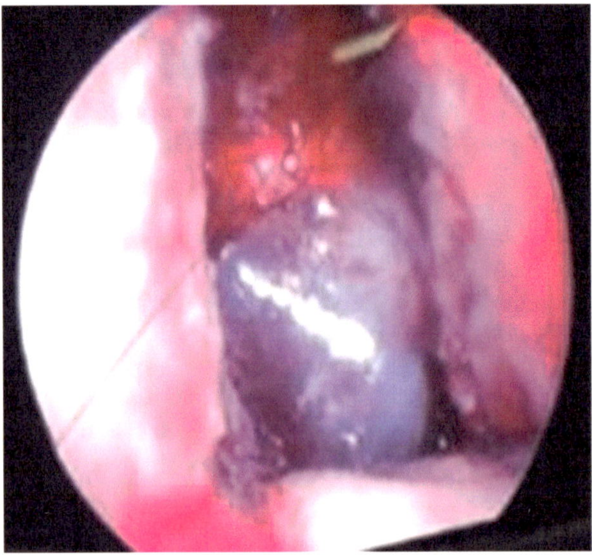

Figure 4.
Reconstruction of skull base defect.

Removal of tumor: Endoscopic bipolar diathermy was applied for the devascularization of tumor from the base. The tumor was removed by standard microsurgery technique under endoscopic view with identification of tumor arachnoid interphase (**Figure 3**).

Closure of skull defect: Skull base defect reconstruction was done with fat, fascia lata, Haddad flap, and reinforced with platelet-rich fibrin. In some cases, we used middle turbinate as a vascularized flap (**Figure 4**).

4. Results

4.1 Demography and Preop radiological findings

Table 1 shows the distribution of demography and prep radiological findings. Most of the patients were in the age group 31–40 years. There was female preponderance.

In neuroimaging, the tuberculum sella location was in seven cases, planum sphenoidale was in four cases, and the TS-PS region was in one case. All optic canal (OC) involvement and internal carotid artery (ICA) encasement cases arose from tuberculum sella meningioma (**Figure 5**).

4.2 Resection status

Figure 6 shows the distribution resection status of the tumor. Complete resection of the tumor could be achieved in eight cases and incomplete resection in four cases (cases 2, 3, 4, and 8).

Figure 7 illustrates the post-op complete resection status of the tumor.

Case no	Age (year)	Sex	Radiological location
1	31	F	TS
2	35	M	TS; OC involvement; ICA encasement
3	36	F	TS; OC involvement
4	38	M	TS + PS
5	45	M	TS
6	48	F	PS;
7	50	F	PS;
8	52	M	TS; OC involvement
9	57	F	PS
10	58	F	TS
11	65	M	TS
12	72	F	PS

Table 1.
Demography and Preop radiological findings.

4.3 Ophthalmological outcome

The outcome of visual disturbances revealed, that there was improvement of vision in six cases, constant vision in four cases, and deterioration of vision in two cases (**Figures 8** and **9**).

4.4 Post-op complications

The post of complications were nasal complications including encrustation, synechiae, and anosmia found in five cases, cerebrospinal fluid (CSF) leak in two cases, and tumor recurrence in two cases. There was Diabetes Insipidus (DI) in one case (**Table 2**).

5. Discussion

Tuberculum sella and planum sphenoidale meningiomas are challenging anterior skull base tumors due to their treacherous anatomical relationship with neurovascular and endocrine structures. These lesions give rise to an early visual pathology with relatively slow progression. They may remain undiagnosed for longer periods of time because tumour-related other symptoms are missing or are subtle [7]. Surgical removal by craniotomy may result in traction injury to the visual apparatus, hypothalamic structures and there may be trouble in skull base hemostasis. On the other hand, the endonasal route can avoid these technical issues by good visualization from the bottom with control of the skull base vascular supply of the tumor. In the study, Ottenhausen et al., have shown that patients treated through extended endoscopic approaches might benefit from better rates of complete surgical resection, and visual

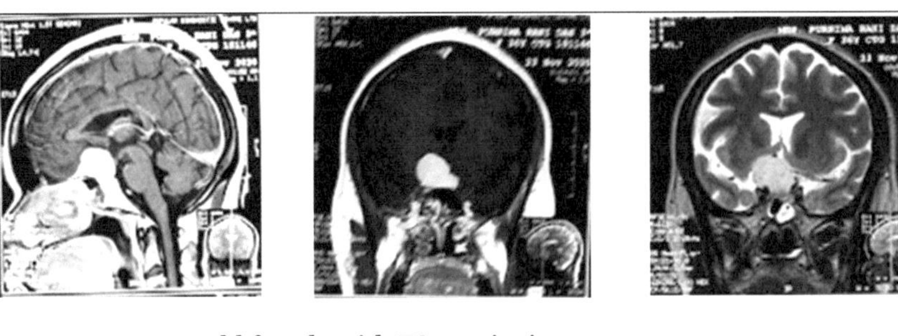

Case 1: A 31- year-old female with TS meningioma.

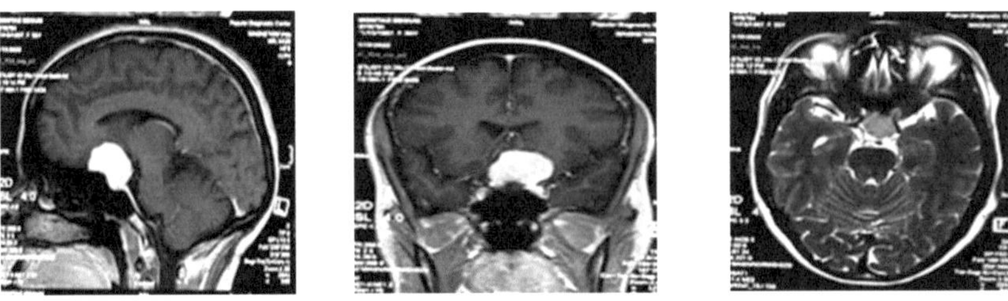

Case 2: A 35- year-old male having TS meningioma with OC involvement and left ICA encasement.

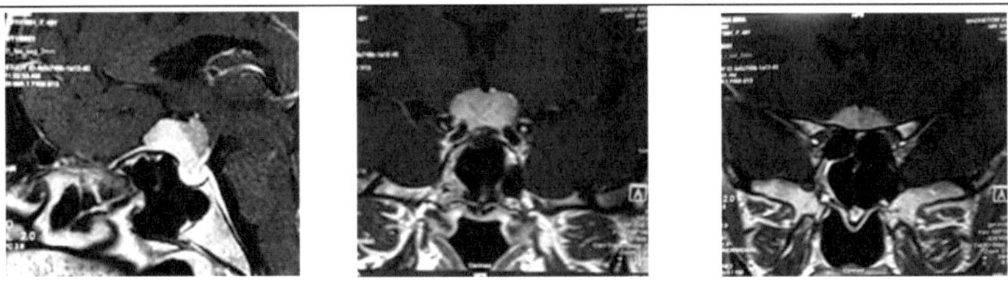

Case 3: A 36- year-old female having TS+PS complex meningioma.

Figure 5.
Radiological illustration of cases.

outcome with preservation of olfaction, less CSF leakage with visual improvement [8]. Both mastery of conventional operative techniques and thorough endoscopic skills are essential for consistent, effective, and safe surgical performance [9].

Although there is some limitation of the surgical corridor through the endoscopic endonasal transsphenoidal approach, the removal of the medial portion of the lesser wing and anterior clinoid process increase the exposure and surgical freedom of the expanded endonasal approach [10].

There are cases described in the literature of tuberculum sellae meningiomas misinterpreted as pituitary macroadenomas, but this was not the case in our study [11].

Out of twelve cases operated, six cases presented an improvement of the visual acuity while in four cases the visual acuity remained stable, overall, this resulted in a stabilization of the preoperative visual acuity in over 83.33% of the treated cases, a percentage that is in accordance with endoscopic resection presented in the literature [12, 13]. In our study, TS meningiomas encasing and displacing the optic apparatus had a poor visual outcome.

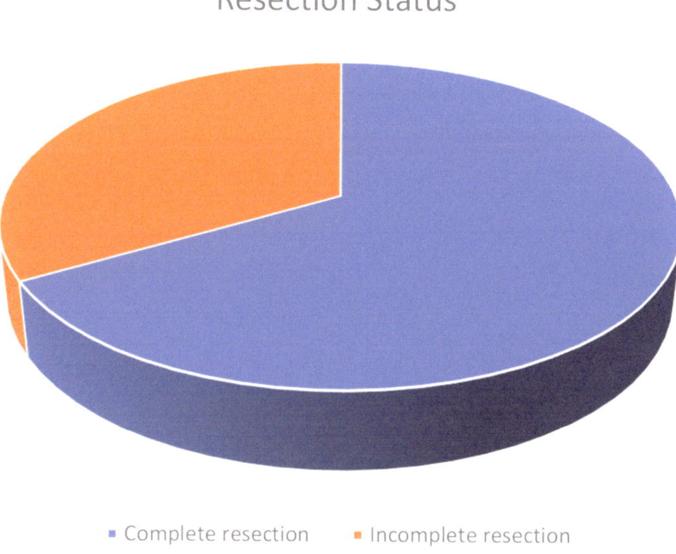

Figure 6.
Distribution of resection status.

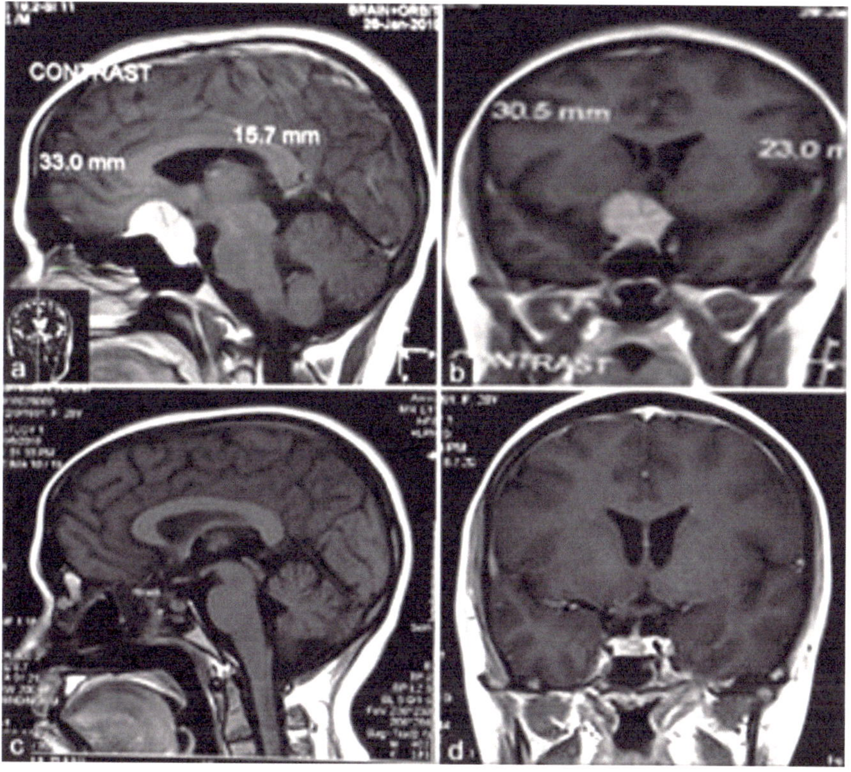

Figure 7.
Radiological illustration of a case of a tuberculum-planum meningioma, preoperative (a and b) and postoperative (c and d).

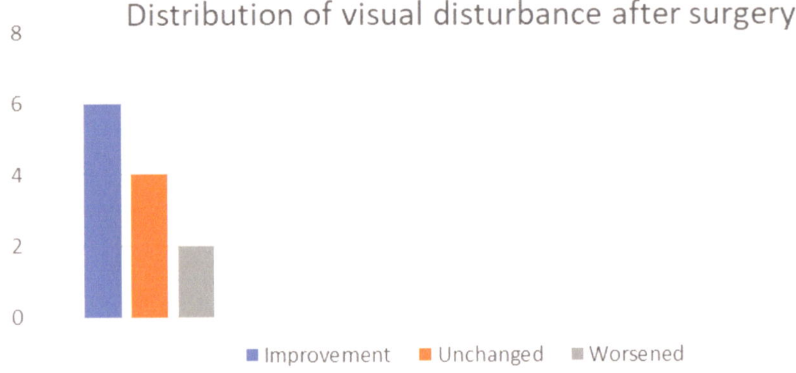

Figure 8.
Distribution of outcome of visual disturbances.

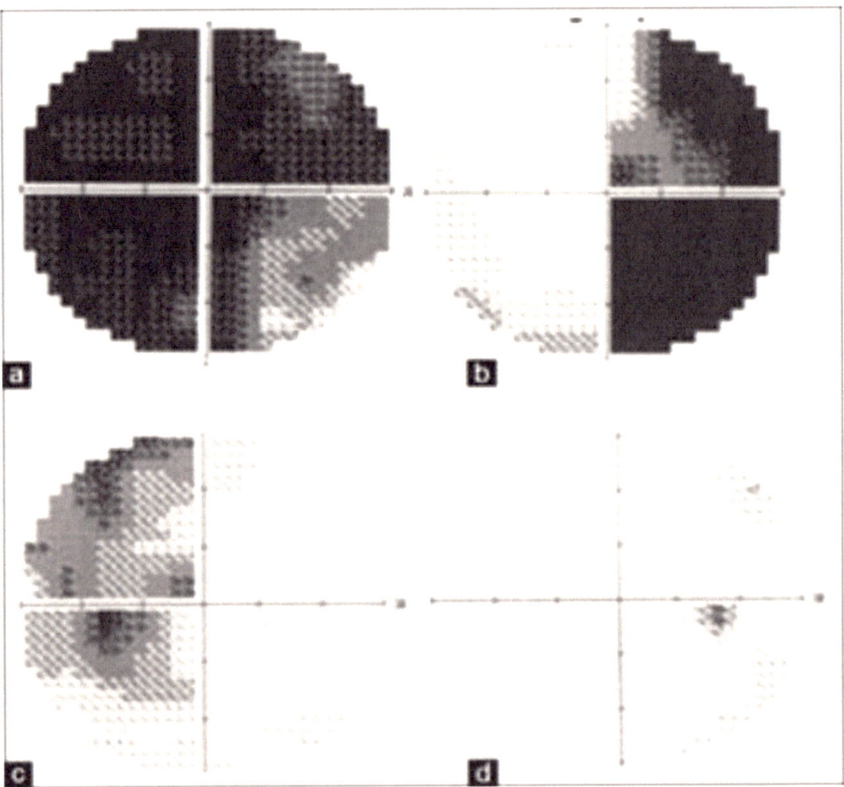

Figure 9.
Ophthalmological illustration, preoperative (a and b), and postoperative (c and d).

Complete resection of the tumor was achieved in 66.67% (12/8) of cases, which is well between the described 56–100% margins found in the literature [13]. Incomplete resection was found in those cases which extended into the optic canal and encasement of vascular structures.

Case no	Complications	Management
1	Nasal encrustation	Nasal wash
2	DI, Tumor recurrence	Transient DI resolved with vasopressin. Tumor recurrence—stable with follow-up scan
3	Tumor recurrence	Revision surgery
4	CSF Rhinorrhoea, Anosmia	Conservative
5		
6	Nasal encrustation	Nasal wash
7		
8	Tumor recurrence	Follow up
9		
10		
11	Anosmia	Assurance
12	Nasal synechiae	Functional endoscopic sinus surgery

Table 2.
Distribution of post-op complications with case distribution.

CSF leak occurred in one case and was managed conservatively. The lower incidence may be due to multilayer closure with vascularized nasoseptal flap.

Nasal complication with anosmia was found in two cases due to extensive dissection of olfactory mucosa for better exposure.

Tumor recurrences occurred in two cases. We believe this is due to the relatively small number of patients included in the study.

6. Conclusion

This study concludes that endoscopic endonasal transsphenoidal resection of TS-PS meningiomas is feasible. This surgical option can provide good tumor clearance, visual improvement, and less complications. This small series does not reflect the standardization of this technique, so larger case series are recommended.

Conflicts of interest

There are no conflicts of interest.

Author details

Md Al Amin Salek*, Rukun Uddin Chowdhury, Ahmed-Ul-Mursalin Chaudhury, Amir Alim, Abdul Hye Manik, Hasnain Faisal, Shamantha Afreen, Nwoshin Jahan and Rajib Sahriar
Department of Neurosurgery, Combined Military Hospital Dhaka, Bangladesh

*Address all correspondence to: salek1972@yahoo.com

References

[1] Chi JH, McDermott MW. Tuberculum sellae meningiomas. Neurosurgical Focus. 2003;**14**:e6

[2] Fernandez-Miranda JC, Pinheiro-Nieto C, Gardner PA, Snyderman CH. Endoscopic endonasal approach for a tuberculum sellae meningioma. Journal of Neurosurgery. 2012;**32**(Suppl):E8

[3] Fahlbusch R, Schott W. Pterional surgery of meningiomas of the tuberculum sellae and planum sphenoidale: Surgical results with special consideration of ophthalmological and endocrinological outcomes. Journal of Neurosurgery. 2002;**96**:235-243

[4] Salek MAA, Faisal MH, Manik MAH, Choudhury AU, Chowdhury RU, Islam MA. Endoscopic endonasal transsphenoidal approach for resection of tuberculum sella and planum sphenoidale meningiomas: A snapshot of our institutional experience. Asian Journal of Neurosurgery. 2020;**15**(1):22-25

[5] Waleed A, Mohamed E, Salem Z, Kamal M. Endoscope-assisted transcranial surgery for anterior skull base meningiomas. Mini-invasive Surgery. 2020;**2020**. DOI: 10.20517/2574-1225.2020.75

[6] Jallo GI, Benjamin V. Tuberculum sellae meningiomas: Microsurgical anatomy and surgical technique. Neurosurgery. 2002;**51**:1432-1439

[7] Ottenhausen M, Banu MA, Placantonakis DG, Tsiouris AJ, Khan OH, Anand VK, et al. Endoscopic endonasal resection of suprasellar meningiomas: The importance of case selection and experience in determining extent of resection, visual improvement, and complications. World Neurosurgery. 2014;**82**:442-449

[8] Krause DE, Grybauskas VT, Friedman M. Instruments and equipment for endoscopic sinus surgery. Otolaryngologic Clinics of North America. 1989;**22**(4):703-711

[9] Di Somma A, Torales J, Cavallo LM, Pineda J, Solari D, Gerardi RM, et al. Defining the lateral limits of the endoscopic endonasal transtuberculum transplanum approach: Anatomical study with pertinent quantitative analysis. Journal of Neurosurgery. 2018;**130**:848-846

[10] Fatemi N, Dusick JR, de Paiva Neto MA, Malkasian D, Kelly DF. Endonasal versus supraorbital keyhole removal of craniopharyngiomas and tuberculum sellae meningiomas. Neurosurgery. 2009;**64**:269-284

[11] Bander ED, Singh H, Ogilvie CB, Cusic RC, Pisapia DJ, Tsiouris AJ, et al. Endoscopic endonasal versus transcranial approach to tuberculum sellae and planum sphenoidale meningiomas in a similar cohort of patients. Journal of Neurosurgery. 2018;**128**:40-48

[12] Kitano M, Taneda M, Nakao Y. Postoperative improvement in visual function in patients with tuberculum sellae meningiomas: Results of the extended transsphenoidal and transcranial approaches. Journal of Neurosurgery. 2007;**107**:337-346

[13] López F, Suárez V, Costales M, Rodrigo JP, Suárez C, Llorente JL. Endoscopic endonasal approach for the treatment of anterior skull base tumours. Acta Otorrinolaringológica Española. 2012;**63**:339-347

Chapter 4

Reconstruction of Scalp and Forehead Defects

Deepak Krishna, Rahul Dubepuria, Manal M. Khan and Amit Agrawal

Abstract

The scalp and forehead are a specialized area of skin that protects the skull, and they differ based on color, long hair, and esthetic appearance. The skull bone is a subcutaneous bone that gets exposed after trauma, electric burn, infection, and following scalp tumor excision. Long-term exposure to the skull may lead to life-threatening complications, such as brain abscess or meningitis. Options of coverage of scalp defects based on its location, depth, size, need for radiation, surrounding skin condition, and esthetic appearance. Partial or complete removal of skull bone may be required, depending on the bone's condition and the disease's nature. Options for cranioplasty rely on the size, location of the skull defect, and need for radiation. Most scalp defects can be managed with local scalp flaps with or without skin grafting at the donor site. Local flaps provide esthetic results because of their architectural similarity to the recipient site.

Keywords: scalp and forehead reconstruction, scalp flap, scalp defect, cranioplasty, bipedicle scalp flap

1. Introduction

The scalp and forehead are multilayered structures covering the skull. Physically, it protects the cranium from external forces, controlling the temperature, and is esthetically vital due to the presence of long hairs and involvement in facial expression. Defects in this region may be superficial, leaving intact pericranium, for example, trauma, avulsion injuries, thermal burn, skin infection, and following excision of benign skin lesions [1, 2]. Avulsion injury of the scalp is common in female workers because of long hair [3]. The high vascularity of the pericranium allows coverage with a skin graft in the superficial defects. Deep wounds usually occur after electric contact burn, excision of malignant skin tumors, high forced avulsion injuries with exposure of skull bone, or even loss of bone segment with exposure of dura or brain. Reconstruction of these deep wounds is challenging for plastic surgeons, neurosurgeons, and oncosurgeons. Because of the thick galea layer, even primary closure of small scalp defects is difficult, so surgeons should have experience with all reconstructive procedures [4]. Reconstructive options for coverage include primary closure, secondary healing, skin grafting, local flaps, regional flaps, tissue expansion, and free tissue transfer [5]. Essential factors, such as defect size, location, components, need for radiation, hairy or non-hairy nature of skin, surrounding tissue condition, and the potential for hairline distortion should be considered while selecting the coverage technique [6–8]. In addition, the basic knowledge of vascularity, innervation, components, and skin mobility in different areas is necessary while dealing with tissue loss in this region. Priority should be reconstruction with local flap with primary closure of donor site or grafted donor site placed in the less cosmetic area, resulting in a better esthetic outcome. Free tissue transfer is a time-consuming procedure and carries higher donor site morbidity than local flaps, unsuitable for high-risk patients.

2. Anatomy of the scalp and forehead

The scalp and forehead are usually considered a single unit but differ in color, texture, esthetic subunit, hair growth length, and pattern. The layers of tissue are almost similar in both areas except the galea layer of the scalp, replaced by the frontalis muscle in the forehead. The knowledge of vascular and nerve supply is helpful during the planning of reconstructive techniques without damaging the motor and sensory supply, especially in the forehead area, and identification of the recipient's vessel for free tissue transfer.

2.1 Scalp

The scalp is formed by five layers, which can be remembered by the mnemonic SCALP: Skin, subcutaneous fat, galea aponeurotica, loose areolar tissue, and pericranium. Scalp skin is thickest in the body and carries long hairs, posing difficulties while reconstructing with similar tissue. The subcutaneous fat layer contains the hair follicles, blood vessels, and fibrous septa, which connect the skin to the galea. Any dissection superficial to galea causes damage to hair follicles and excessive bleeding. Galea aponeurotica connects the frontalis muscle anteriorly and the occipital muscle posteriorly. Laterally, it continues as temporoparietal fascia and is confluent with the superficial musculoaponeurotic system of the face. Loose areolar tissue beneath galea aponeurotica allows the avascular plane for dissection. The temporal branch of the facial nerve runs in the temporoparietal fascia and gets protected while raising the bicoronal flap in this loose areolar plane [9]. The pericranium is the deepest layer covering the skull bones except at the temporal region, where it is fused with the deep temporal fascia, which covers the temporal muscle. The calvaria comprises eight bones formed by intramembranous ossification (frontal, paired parietal, and paired temporal bones) and endochondral ossification (occipital, ethmoid, and sphenoid bones). These bones are fused by four sutures named metopic, coronal, sagittal, and lambdoid. The calvaria has three layers: an outer table, a diploic space, and an inner table. The superior sagittal sinus is the most superficial sinus that runs in the midline under the sagittal suture and needs care while doing bony debridement in this region.

2.2 Forehead

The forehead is the upper part of the face, bounded superiorly and laterally by the anterior hairline and inferiorly by the supraorbital margin. It contains the paired frontalis muscle, which elevates the eyebrows and blends with the procerus medially, the corrugator centrally, and the orbicularis oculi laterally. A temporal branch of the facial nerve innervates the frontalis and corrugator muscles, whereas the deep buccal branch of the facial nerve innervates the procerus.

2.3 Arterial supply

The scalp and forehead supply blood from paired supraorbital, supratrochlear, superficial temporal, posterior auricular, and occipital arteries. Supraorbital and supratrochlear arise from the ophthalmic artery, the first branch of the internal carotid artery, and other arteries are branches of the external carotid artery.

2.4 Venous drainage

Supraorbital and supratrochlear veins form the angular vein and drain into the facial vein. The superficial temporal and maxillary veins form the retromandibular vein, which divides into anterior and posterior divisions. The anterior division combines with the facial vein and includes a common facial vein, which drains into the internal jugular vein. The posterior division combines with the posterior auricular vein and forms the external jugular vein, which drains into the subclavian vein. The occipital vein drains into the suboccipital plexus.

2.5 Sensory supply

The paired sensory nerves of the scalp and forehead include supratrochlear (V1), supraorbital (V1), zygomaticotemporal (V2), auriculotemporal (V3), lesser occipital (C2–C3), and greater occipital (C2) nerves. The supraorbital and supratrochlear nerves supply the forehead and frontoparietal region of the scalp. The zygomatico-temporal nerve supplies the region laterals to the brow and the temporal area of the scalp up to the temporal line. The auriculotemporal nerve supplies the lateral scalp region, and the greater and lesser occipital nerves supply the occipital region.

2.6 Lymphatic drainage

The part anterior to the ear drains into preauricular and parotid lymph nodes, whereas the part posterior to the ear drains into postauricular and occipital lymph nodes.

2.7 Etiology

The scalp and forehead defects usually arise after traumatic injury, including avulsion, tumor resection, congenital, electric, thermal burn, infection, and post-radiation [10]. Trends of traumatic injuries are increasing due to the rise in roadside accidents and workplace injuries. Total or partial scalp avulsion injuries are more common in females because of long hairs [3]. The scalp and forehead are also common skin cancer sites because they are directly exposed to sunlight [5]. Many benign and congenital pathologies require excision followed by reconstruction. High voltage electric burn over the scalp is common in developing countries, causing exposure of skull bone. Radiation following tumor excision of the scalp or brain causes dehiscence of the suture line and ulceration, even exposure to implants [11].

2.8 Esthetic consideration of the scalp and forehead

The scalp is a single esthetic unit having thick hair-bearing skin demarcated by the anterior and temporal hairline. Preserving the hairline is a must while doing local flaps to cover the scalp and forehead defects. The direction of hair growth varies in the different anatomical areas of the scalp, so incisions should be planned parallel to them, and minimum use of electrocautery to prevent visible scarring. The frontal, parietal, and vertex are more of a cosmetic concern than the temporal and occipital areas. Historically, the forehead has been subdivided into one central unit, two temporal units posterior to the anterior temporal crest, and two eyebrow units along the supraorbital rims. Recently, the forehead has been subdivided into paramedian, lateral, and lateral temporal subunits [12].

2.9 Assessment of the defect and treatment planning

A detailed history and local examination are essential before selecting a reconstructive technique. Associated medical conditions, such as diabetes, hypertension, smoking, coronary artery disease, and asthma, should be assessed along with previous surgery and radiation history. In clinical examination, defect size, location, depth, surrounding skin condition, hairy or non-hairy nature of skin at the defect site, and potential for hairline distortion should be kept in mind. Defects following trauma and benign lesion excision are primarily superficial and can be managed with skin grafting if not able to closed with similar local tissue. Oncological resection is usually deep and requires the removal of bone, which may be reconstructed immediately along with a flap cover or in the second stage. Long-standing exposure of skull bone in electric contact burn also necessitates the removal of partial or complete bone followed by flap coverage [13]. Dural defects must be repaired with artificial patches or a non-vascularized fascial graft. Small defects at the forehead and scalp are manageable with primary closure or local flaps. Mobility of skin and availability of arc of rotation is

Wound characteristics	Consideration
Location of the defect	Forehead Central Lateral Scalp Frontal Parietal Vertex Temporal Occipital Combined
Size of defect	Small (<4 cm^2) Medium (4–50 cm^2) Large (50–200 cm^2) Very large (>200 cm^2)
Depth	Subcutis Pericranium Bone/implant Dura Brain
Surrounding structure	Nearby scarring Hairy or non-hairy skin Hairline and brow position

Table 1.
Factors determining selection of graft.

less in the central region, which necessitates the closure of the medium-sized defects by a double rotation flap compared to the peripheral area, where a single rotation flap can cover. A skin graft is acceptable for the defect at the non-hairy scalp. Coverage of large scalp defect with a transposition flap necessitates skin grafting at the donor site, which should be kept in a less esthetic place (temporal, occipital) so that nearby long hairs can cover the skin-grafted area. In avulsion injuries, you may sometimes find an injured vascular pedicle, necessitating using a vein graft or arterio-venous loop to use recipient vessels outside the trauma zone for reimplantation or free tissue transfer (**Table 1**).

3. Reconstructive options

3.1 Primary closure

The scalp wound up to 3 cm in diameter is considered amenable to primary closure [14]. The galeal layer is a rigid structure with limited mobility, so wide skin undermining is required to close the defect primarily in a tension-free manner. Galea scoring perpendicular to the line of maximum tension and parallel to the subaponeurotic blood vessel is also helpful in facilitating tension-free closure [15, 16].

The forehead skin is mobile, and slight undermining in the subcutaneous plane results in the primary closure of the small defects. The horizontal scar along the natural crease is cosmetic appealing but has the risk of upliftment of brow position. Vertical closure avoids this problem but decreases the distance between eyebrows when tried in the glabellar region. The Limberg flap maintains the inter-eyebrow distance, transposing the nearby skin at the defect site (**Figure 1**). Linear closure after elliptical excision has a long scar, which can be avoided using "M" plasty.

3.2 Secondary healing

Healing by secondary intention can be allowed for very small scalp defects without exposure to the bone in a hairless area [14]. However, most reconstructive surgeons do not consider this method as it causes bald scars. Superficial burns and abrasions usually heal by secondary intension, but daily dressing is needed for an extended period. Conservatively managed post-traumatic and burn wounds over the forehead produce a shift of hairline and eyebrow position due to wound contraction (**Figure 2**). The upward shift of the eyebrow may pull the eyelid tissue. A vacuum-assisted closure device helps to fasten the wound contraction in chronic nonhealing wounds with continuous discharge (**Figure 3**).

3.3 Skin grafting

Skin grafting may be considered for large-sized defects at the forehead and scalp area, which cannot be covered by local flaps with primary closure of the flap donor site. The lateral forehead, temporal, and occipital regions are of less cosmetic importance (**Figure 4**), and defects in this region can be resurfaced with skin grafting. Preservation of pericranium is a prerequisite for skin grafting. The disadvantage of this procedure are scar alopecia, instability in the long term, and not suitable for radiation therapy. These skin-grafted areas can be replaced by expanded flaps from nearby areas later for cosmetic reasons. Skin grafting suits patients with comorbidities

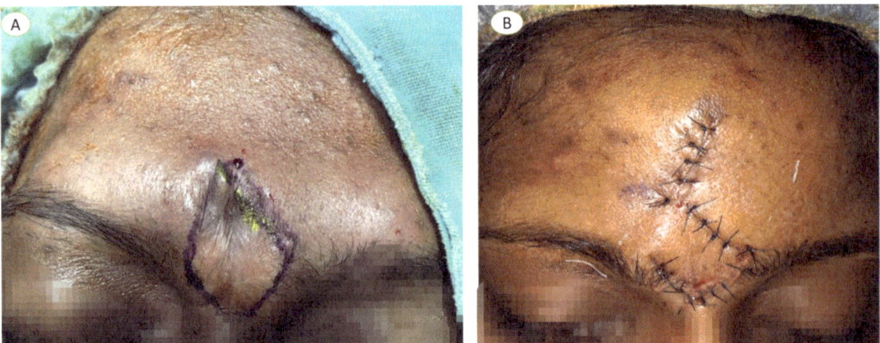

Figure 1.
A. Scarring over forehead following Bindi application; B. Excision of scar and coverage with Limberg flap.

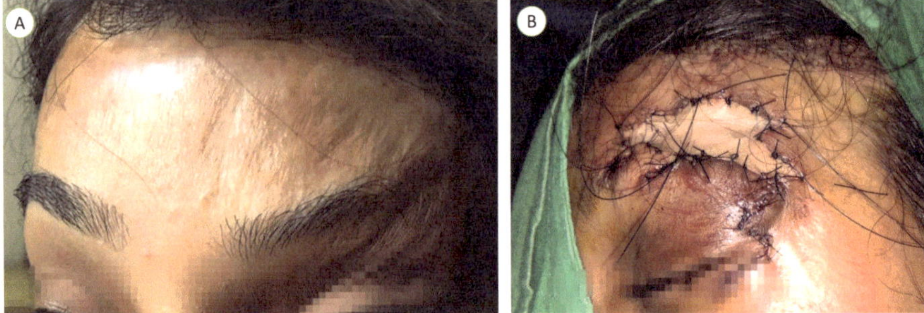

Figure 2.
A. Postburn scarring on the left side of forehead causing eyebrow and lid upward pull; B. Correction of lid deformity by Z plasty at lateral canthal region and skin grafting after the release of brow pull.

who can not tolerate major surgeries. A free split-thickness skin graft can be done after drilling down to the diploic layer of bone to improve the granulation process for coverage of broad defects more significant than 100 cm^2 with loss of pericranium when other options are not feasible [17]. The use of a dermal regenerative template has also been described after removing the external table to improve the cosmetic outcome and durability of the graft [18, 19]. However, the increased cost of treatment and risk of infection are there. Combined vacuum-assisted closure dressing and a dermal regenerative template can improve wound beds when vital structures are exposed to scalp wounds [20].

3.4 Local flaps

Local scalp tissue arrangement can cover small- to medium-sized defects with donor area closure. Defects up to 50 cm^2 in the peripheral (temporal, parietal, and occipital) region allow coverage with a single rotation flap (**Figure 5**) because making a wide arc of rotation is possible [13]. Planning of double opposing rotation flaps (**Figure 6**) is needed for the similar-sized defects at the vertex regions. The arc of the rotation flap must be marked at the periphery four to five times the defect margin, ensuring primary closure of the donor area. The rotation flap requires a wide undermining and long incision and is time-consuming compared to the transposition flap. Therefore, it should be avoided in unstable patients. Injecting an adrenaline solution

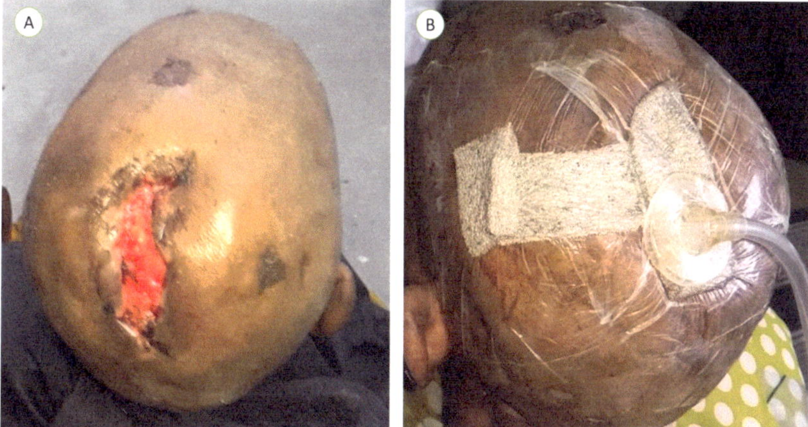

Figure 3.
A. Infected wound over the scalp with recurrent dehiscence; B. Promoting secondary healing by vacuum-assisted closure device.

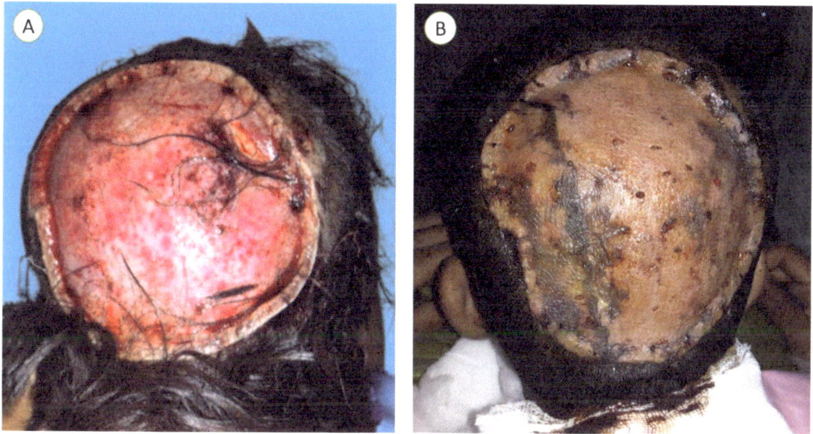

Figure 4.
A. Scalp avulsion injury over the occipital region with a defect size of 12 × 10 cm; B. Skin graft application over intact pericranium.

of 1:200,000 dilution at the marking site reduces blood loss, and the flap is elevated in the avascular plane with the preservation of the pericranium. Backcut at the pivot point toward the flap base and galea scoring is advisable for tension-free closure.

The central forehead defects need coverage with an O-T flap with a transverse incision along the hairline when defects are located at the middle and upper parts (**Figure 7**). For defects at the lower part of the forehead, transverse incisions need to be made just above the eyebrow to avoid approximation of the medial end of the eyebrows. Lateral forehead defects can be covered with a worthen flap [21] or temporoparietal fascia flap with an overlying skin graft (**Figure 8**). The temporoparietal fascia flap has a wide arc of rotation from the postauricular region to the lateral forehead. This fascial flap is supplied by a temporal branch of the superficial temporal artery, which runs just under the surface of the fascia. The plane of dissection between skin and fascia is demanding; too superficial dissection and excessive use of

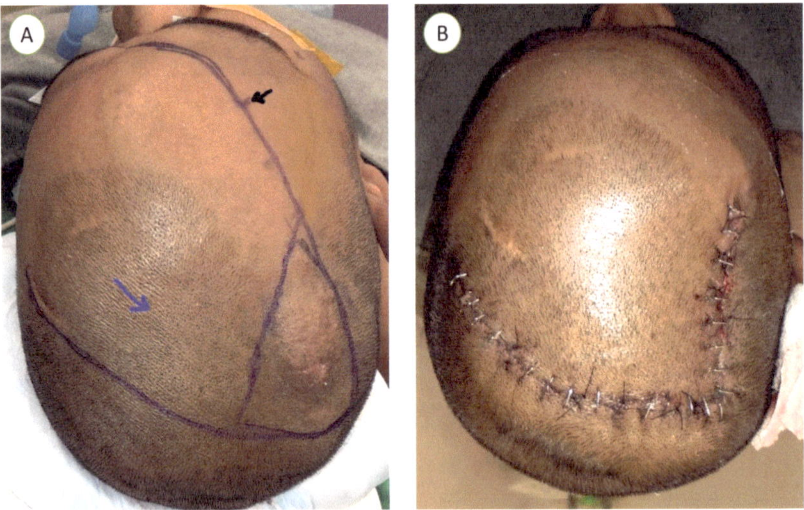

Figure 5.
A. Benign skin lesion at right parietal region; B. Excision of the lesion and coverage with a single rotation flap.

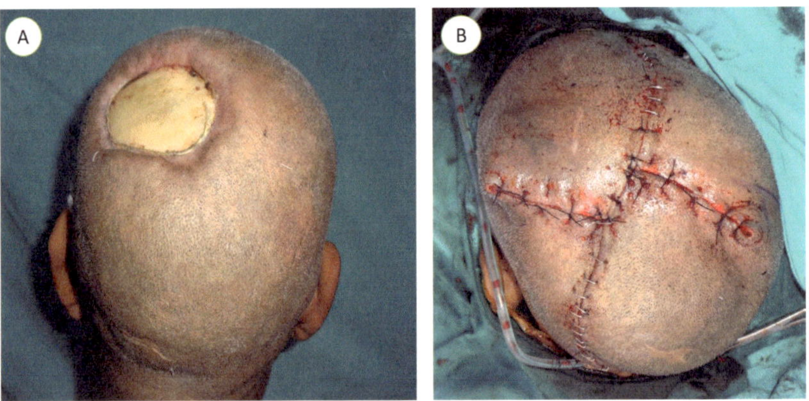

Figure 6.
A. Exposed skull bone following post-electric contact burn; B. Debridement and coverage with double rotation flap.

electrocautery may result in postoperative alopecia. Temporoparietal fascia with the temporal skin strip can be used for eyebrow reconstruction where the skin is scarred and not suitable for hair grafting (**Figure 9**). The temporalis muscle, supplied by the deep temporal artery, is a valuable flap for resurfacing the orbital cavity following exenteration. A piece of bone can be elevated along with the temporalis muscle, with its deep fascial extension used in various facial reanimation procedures.

There are large defects where the donor site cannot be closed using a rotation flap; a transposition flap is suggested. The length of the transposition flap should be from the flap's pivot point to the defect's farthest point with a length-to-width ratio of up to 1:1 to 1:3 with the named vessel at the pedicle base. When the length-to-width percentage increases more than 1:3, or the flap distal margin crosses the midline, planning a bipedicle flap is advisable to increase the flap's vascularity. The bipedicle fronto-occipital (**Figure 10**) and temporo-temporal (**Figure 11**) flaps are supplied

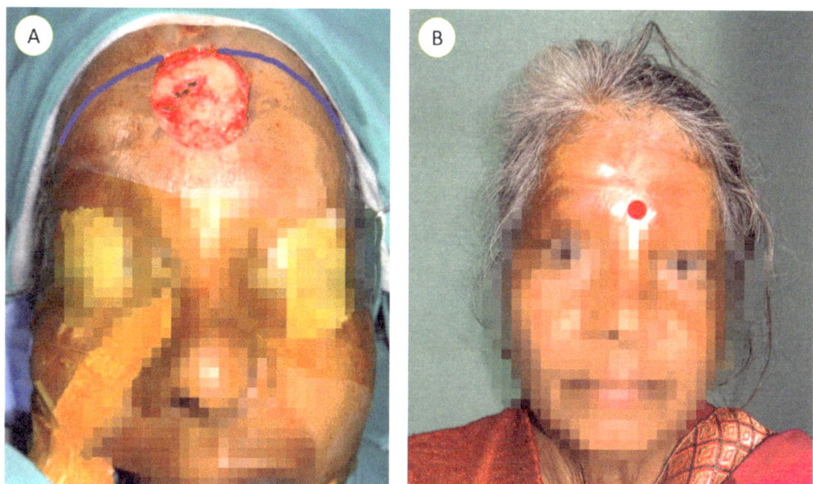

Figure 7.
A. Mid forehead defect of size 5 × 5 cm following excision of an unstable scar; B. Coverage with O-T flap.

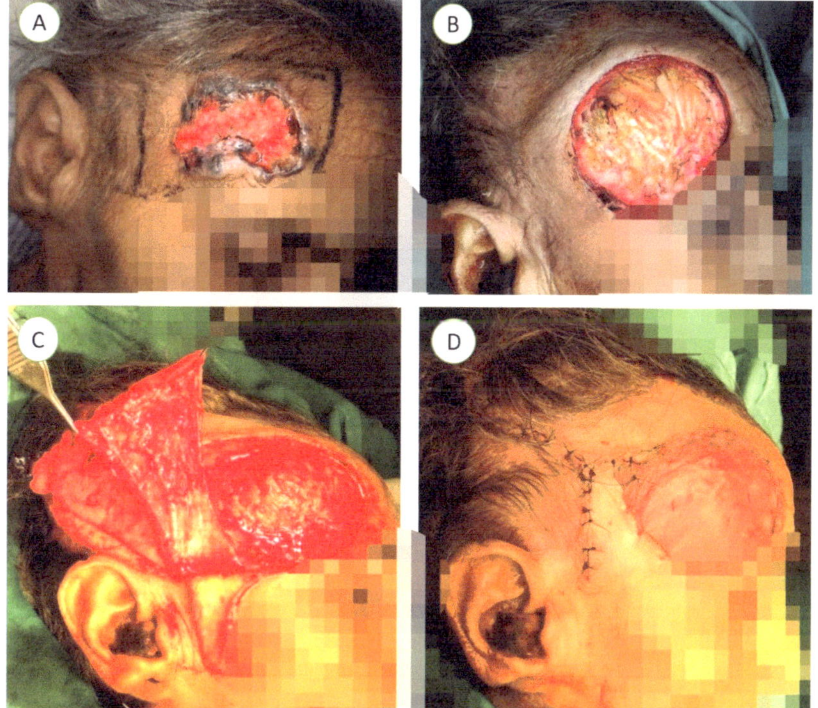

Figure 8.
A. Basal cell carcinoma at right lateral forehead; B. After excision of the lesion defects size of 7 × 6 cm and exposed bone; C. Raised temporoparietal fascia flap; D. Coverage of the defect with fascial flap and overlying skin graft.

by named vessels at both ends and have a wide coverage scale. The dog ear at the flap base in the transposition flap should not be excised immediately because it would narrow the pedicle and decrease its blood supply. The donor site of the transposition flap

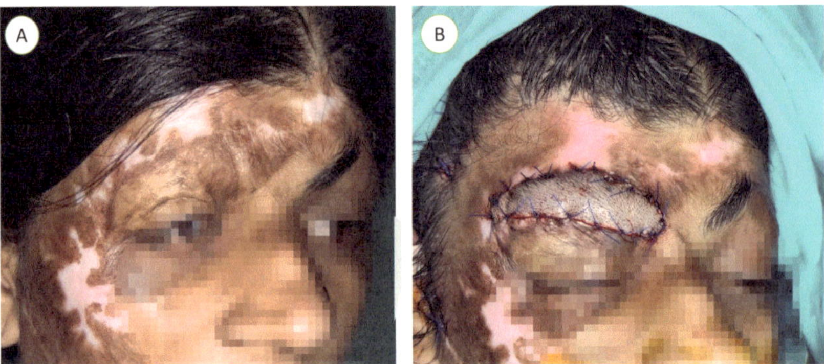

Figure 9.
A. Postburn eyebrow loss with surrounding scarring; B. Brow reconstruction with temporoparietal fasciocutaneous flap.

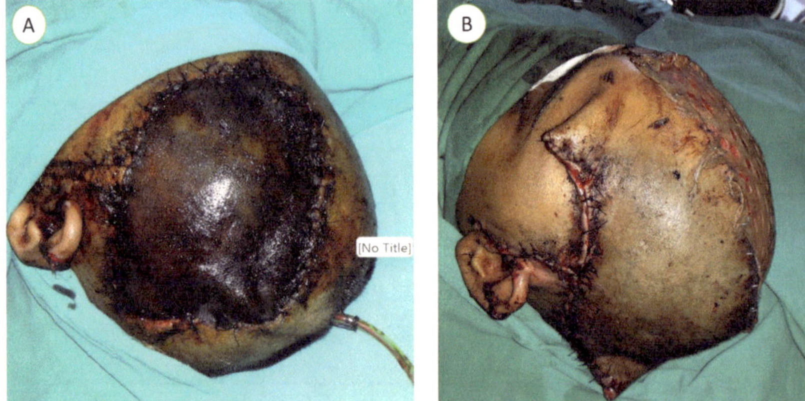

Figure 10.
A. Necrotic scalp skin following avulsion injury left temporoparietal region; B. Debridement and coverage with bipedicle fronto-occipital flap with skin graft at the flap donor site for defect size of 18 × 10 cm.

needs skin grafting. The donor site of the transposition flap at the less cosmetic and bald area (**Figure 12**) provides acceptable results [13].

The galeopericranial, pericranial, and galeal flaps are highly reliable and versatile for anterior skull base defect reconstruction to prevent cerebrospinal fluid leaks and brain herniation [22, 23]. The pericranial flap is routinely used to obliterate the nasofrontal duct following cranialization of the frontal sinus (**Figure 13**). These flaps are designed to have a base toward the defects. They are elevated during the bicoronal flap elevation. Split calvarial bone grafts with pericranial flap have been described for reconstructing large anterior skull base defects.

3.5 Regional flaps

Due to limited reach, the regional flap is restricted to the occipital and lateral forehead regions. Expanded flap from face usually advanced to lateral forehead in managing the postburn scarring. Extended supraclavicular, pectoralis major, and latissimus dorsi flap have been described to cover the lateral face and forehead. A lower trapezius musculocutaneous flap is commonly performed to protect the

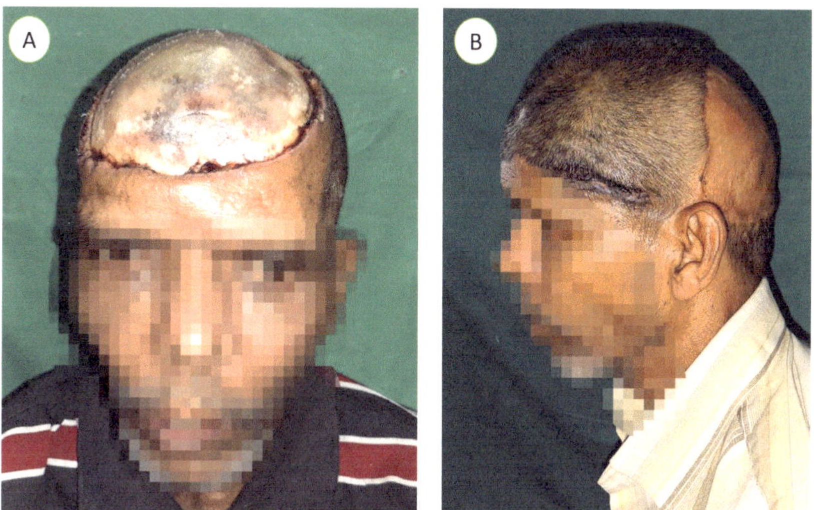

Figure 11.
A. Post-electric contact burns with exposed skull bone at frontoparietal region; B. Defect covered with bipedicle bucket handle flap and skin graft at the flap donor site.

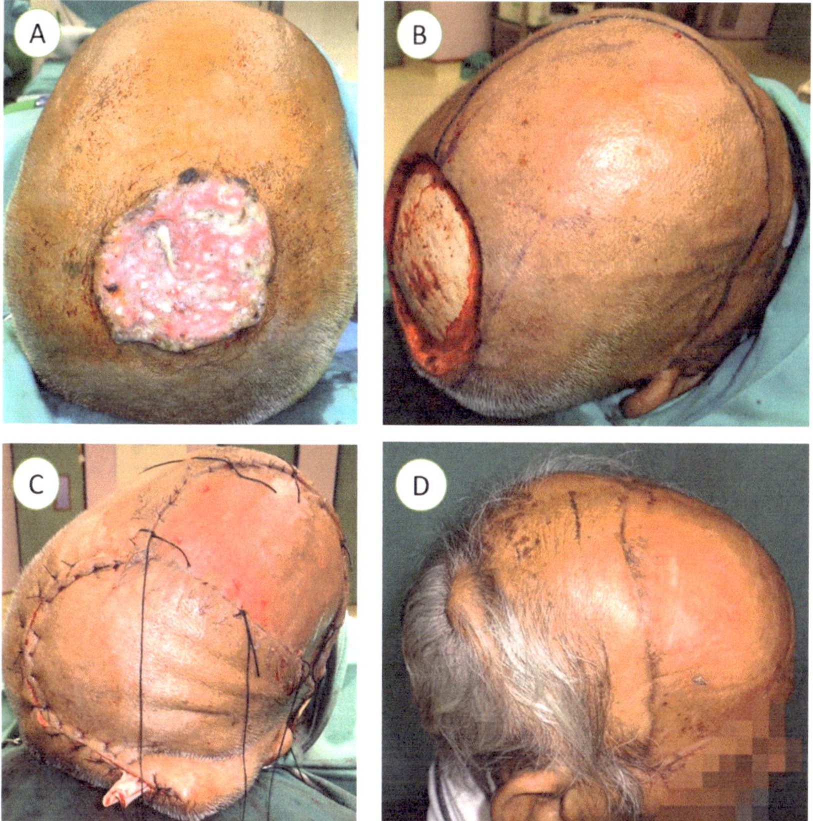

Figure 12.
A. Squamous cell carcinoma on the right parietal region; B. 8 × 8 cm size defect after wide local excision; C. Coverage with transposition flap from the bald area; D. 3 months postoperative result.

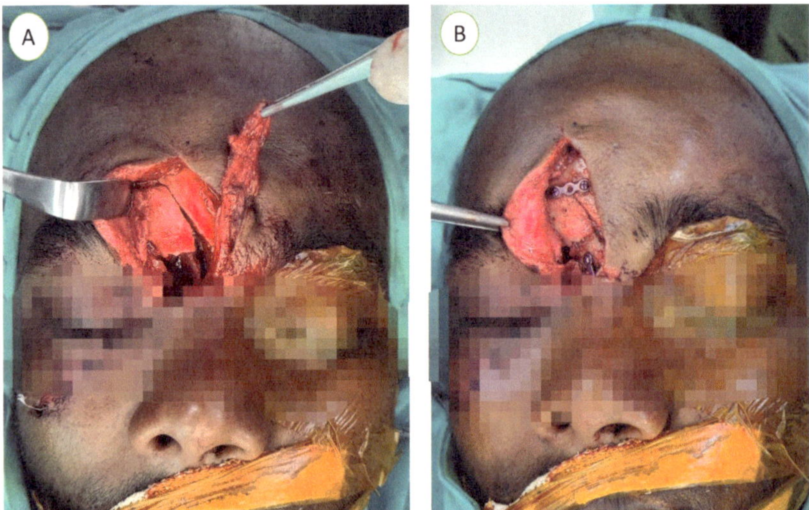

Figure 13.
A. Cranialization of the frontal sinus and elevation of the pericranial flap; B. Fixation of the anterior table after blockage of the nasofrontal duct with pericranial flap.

occipital defects with exposure of bone and implants. These distant pedicle flaps, such as trapezius, pectoralis, and latissimus dorsi myo-cutaneous flaps, are marked on the distal point of flap territory to maximize the reach, which also increases the chances of flap ischemia. Other disadvantages of distant flaps are non-hairy, poor skin color match, thick pedicle, and bulky skin paddle [24].

3.6 Microvascular reconstruction

Local and regional flaps cannot cover extensive scalp defects >200 cm^2 area. In these conditions, free tissue transfer is indicated for the best outcome. Free tissue transfers are mainly required after post-tumor resection with loss of pericranium or calvarial defect with exposed dura. Other indications are extensive avulsion injury and electric contact burn of the scalp and forehead. Latissimus dorsi muscle flap, anterolateral thigh flap, para scapular flap, rectus abdominal flap, radial forearm flap, etc., are some commonly used free flaps for scalp and forehead reconstruction [25–27]. Among the free flaps, muscle flaps with an overlying skin graft are less bulky than fasciocutaneous flaps and provide better contour. Free latissimus dorsi is a workhorse flap in scalp reconstruction (**Figure 14**) with a broader scale of coverage and acceptable donor site morbidity. Fasciocutaneous free flaps are preferred when the calvarial bone is reconstructed using titanium mesh implants because there are no chances of atrophy, scarring, and better postoperative radiation toleration [28]. Fasciocutaneous flaps are also preferred for forehead reconstruction and when secondary cranioplasty is planned. The esthetic outcome of free flaps is lower when compared to local flaps but more than skin grafting.

3.7 Scalp replantation

Scalp replantation is the standard treatment for complete and partial scalp avulsion injury. No other procedure can give results, such as replantation. Loose areolar tissue allows subgaleal dissection during the entrapment of scalp hair in a moving machine. Many times, some parts of the pericranium are also lost. The first patient

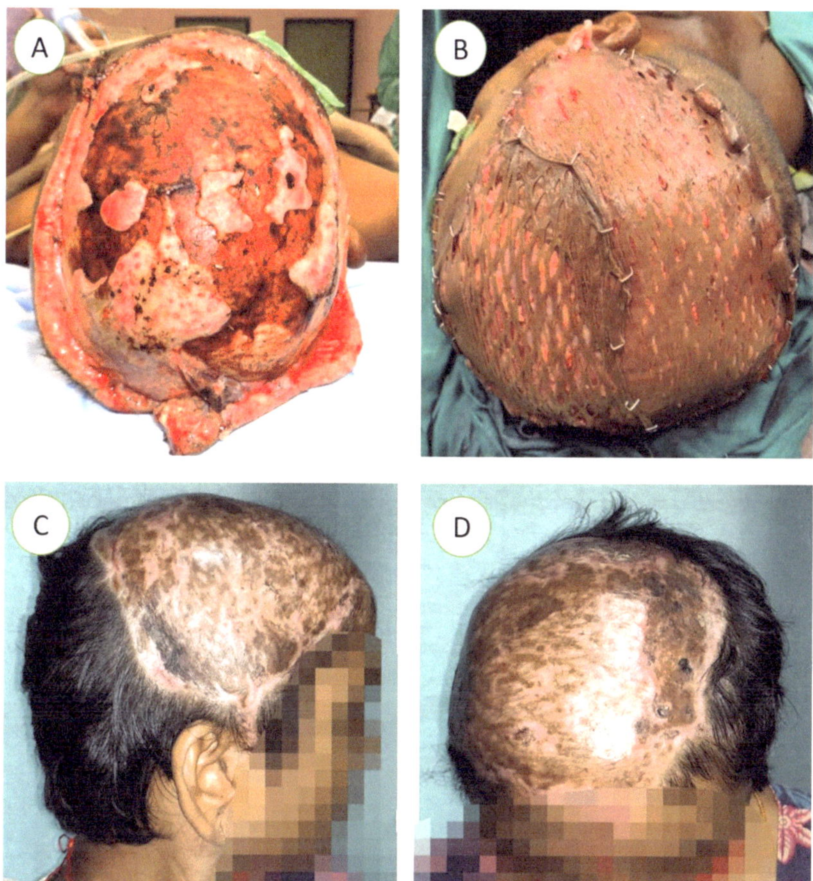

Figure 14.
A. Near total scalp avulsion with exposed skull bone; B. Coverage with free latissimus dorsi muscle flap and overlying skin graft; C and D. 6 months follow-up results.

should be stabilized hemodynamically. If the avulsed part is in good condition, repair of the single artery can survive the whole avulsed skin. Two team approaches can need to work simultaneously to shorten the surgery duration. The superficial temporal artery and vein are the most used recipient vessels for anastomosis. Two veins should be repaired to prevent the risk of venous congestion. A vein graft may be required if recipient vessels are injured. Nerve repair is indicated for recovery of sensation.

3.8 Calvarial reconstruction

The different etiologies of calvarial defects are traumatic loss, post-oncological resection, removal of dead bone, and craniectomy defect following intracranial surgeries. Immediate reconstruction of calvarial defects after craniectomy determined by the size and location of bone defects and expected intracranial pressure. Indications of cranioplasty are protection from trauma, cosmesis, and the putative "syndrome of trephined." Small- to medium-sized bone defects (≤5–7 cm) in cosmetic and pressure-sensitive areas, such as the forehead or occipital region indicate cranioplasty. Morselized bone grafts for small-size defects and calvarial or rib grafts for medium-size defects are advisable [27]. However, large-size bony defects require a vascularized rib graft with a free latissimus dorsi muscle flap cover [29]. But nowadays, titanium mesh is an excellent alternative to autograft in all types of defects. Non-vascularized bone grafts and prosthetic material are not advisable when postoperative radiotherapy is planned. Bone resorption, exposure, and infection are the most common complications following cranioplasty, leading to revision surgery [30].

4. Summary

Local scalp flaps can cover small- to medium-sized scalp and forehead defects. Primary closure of the donor area or skin grafting at a less cosmetic area results in better esthetic outcomes. Large-sized defects, the need for postoperative radiation, and coverage after bony reconstruction indicate free tissue transfer. A single or double rotation flap selection depends on the defect's location and the donor area's availability rather than the size. Single or bipedicle transposition scalp flaps have a wider coverage scale, are less time-consuming, and are advisable in high-risk patients. Debridement of the outer surface of the cranium is needed in long-standing exposed bone or to promote granulation before skin grafting.

Conflict of interest

The authors have no conflicts of interest relevant to this article.

Author details

Deepak Krishna[1*], Rahul Dubepuria[2], Manal M. Khan[1] and Amit Agrawal[3]

1 Department of Burns and Plastic Surgery, All India Institute of Medical Sciences, Bhopal, Madhya Pradesh, India

2 Department of Trauma and Emergency, All India Institute of Medical Sciences, Bhopal, India

3 Department of Neurosurgery, All India Institute of Medical Sciences, Bhopal, India

*Address all correspondence to: deepak.plasticsurg@aiimsbhopal.edu.in

References

[1] TerKonda RP, Sykes JM. Concepts in scalp and forehead reconstruction. Otolaryngologic Clinics of North America. 1997;**30**(4):519-539

[2] Mueller CK, Bader RD, Ewald C, Kalff R, Schultze-Mosgau S. Scalp defect repair: A comparative analysis of different surgical techniques. Annals of Plastic Surgery. 2012;**68**:594-598

[3] Kalra GS, Goil P, Chakotiya PS. Microsurgical reconstruction of major scalp defects following scalp avulsion. Indian Journal of Plastic Surgery. 2013;**46**:486-492

[4] Hoffman JF. Management of scalp defects. Otolaryngologic Clinics of North America. 2001;**34**:571-582. DOI: 10.1016/s0030- 6665(05)70006-2

[5] Costa DJ, Walen S, Varvares M, Walker R. Scalp rotation flap for reconstruction of complex soft tissue defects. Journal of Neurology Surgery B Skull Base. 2016;77:32-37

[6] Grigg R. Forehead and temple reconstruction. Otolaryngologic Clinics of North America. 2001;**34**(3):583-600

[7] Leedy JE, Janis JE, Rohrich RJ. Reconstruction of acquired scalp defects: An algorithmic approach. Plastic and Reconstructive Surgery. 2005;**116**:54e-72e

[8] Desai SC, Sand JP, Sharon JD, Branham G, Nussenbaum B. Scalp reconstruction: An algorithmic approach and systematic review. JAMA Facial Plastic Surgery. 2015;**17**:56-66

[9] Stuzin JM, Wagstrom L, Kawamoto HK, Wolfe SA. Anatomy of the frontal branch of the facial nerve: The significance of the temporal fat pad. Plastic and Reconstructive Surgery. 1989;**83**(2):265-271

[10] Zayakova Y, Stanev A, Mihailov H, Pashaliev N. Application of local axial flaps to scalp reconstruction. Archives of Plastic Surgery. 2013;**40**:564-569

[11] Maqbool T, Binhammer A, Binhammer P, Antonyshyn OM. Risk factors for titanium mesh implant exposure following cranioplasty. The Journal of Craniofacial Surgery. 2018;**29**(5):1181-1186

[12] Seline PC, Siegle RJ. Forehead reconstruction. Dermatologic Clinics. 2005;**23**(1):1-v

[13] Krishna D, Khan MM, Dubepuria R, Chaturvedi G, Cheruvu VPR. Reconstruction of scalp and forehead defects: Options and strategies. Cureus. 2023;**15**(7):e41479. Published 2023 Jul 6

[14] Sokoya M, Misch E, Vincent A, Wang W, Kadakia S, Ducic Y, et al. Free tissue reconstruction of the scalp. Seminars in Plastic Surgery. 2019;**33**:67-71

[15] Lin SJ, Hanasono MM, Skoracki RJ. Scalp and calvarial reconstruction. Seminars in Plastic Surgery. 2008;**22**:281-293

[16] Yaremchuk MJ, O'Sullivan N, Benslimane F. Reversing brow lifts. Aesthetic Surgery Journal. 2007;**27**(4):367-375

[17] Gürlek A, Alaybeyoğlu N, Demir CY, Aydoğan H, Bilen BT, Oztürk A. Aesthetic reconstruction of large scalp defects by sequential tissue expansion without interval. Aesthetic Plastic Surgery. 2004;**28**:245-250

[18] Faulhaber J, Felcht M, Teerling G, Klemke CD, Wagner C, Goerdt S, et al. Long-term results after reconstruction of full-thickness scalp defects with a dermal regeneration template. Journal of the European Academy of Dermatology and Venereology. 2010;**24**:572-577

[19] Goerdt S, Faulhaber J. Removal of the outer table of the skull for reconstruction of full-thickness scalp defects with a dermal regeneration template. Dermatologic Surgery. 2008;**34**:357-363

[20] Ahmed O, Storey CM, Zhang S, Chelly MR, Yeoh MS, Nanda A. Vacuum-assisted closure of necrotic and infected cranial wound with loss of dura mater: A technical note. Surgical Neurology International. 2015;**6**:11

[21] Elbanoby TM, Zidan SM, Elbatawy AM, Aly GM, Sholkamy K. Superficial temporal artery flap for reconstruction of complex facial defects: A new algorithm. Archives of Plastic Surgery. 2018;**45**:118-127

[22] Price JC, Loury M, Carson B, Johns ME. The pericranial flap for reconstruction of anterior skull base defects. The Laryngoscope. 1988;**98**(11):1159-1164

[23] Snyderman CH, Janecka IP, Sekhar LN, Sen CN, Eibling DE. Anterior cranial base reconstruction: Role of galeal and pericranial flaps. The Laryngoscope. 1990;**100**(6):607-614

[24] Denewer A, Khater A, Farouk O, et al. Can we put a simplified algorithm for reconstruction of large scalp defects following tumor resection? World Journal of Surgical Oncology. 2011;**9**:129

[25] Herrera F, Buntic R, Brooks D, Buncke G, Antony AK. Microvascular approach to scalp replantation and reconstruction: A thirty-six year experience. Microsurgery. 2012;**32**:591-597

[26] Lipa JE, Butler CE. Enhancing the outcome of free latissimus dorsi muscle flap reconstruction of scalp defects. Head & Neck. 2004;**26**:46-53

[27] van Driel AA, Mureau MA, Goldstein DP, et al. Aesthetic and oncologic outcome after microsurgical reconstruction of complex scalp and forehead defects after malignant tumor resection: An algorithm for treatment. Plastic and Reconstructive Surgery. 2010;**126**:460-470

[28] Weitz J, Spaas C, Wolff KD, Meyer B, Shiban E, Ritschl LM. A standard algorithm for reconstruction of scalp defects with simultaneous free flaps in an interdisciplinary two-team approach. Frontiers in Oncology. 2019;**9**:1130

[29] Seitz IA, Gottlieb LJ. Reconstruction of scalp and forehead defects. Clinics in Plastic Surgery. 2009;**36**:355-377

[30] Steiner D, Horch RE, Eyüpoglu I, et al. Reconstruction of composite defects of the scalp and neurocraniuma treatment algorithm from local flaps to combined AV loop free flap reconstruction. World Journal of Surgical Oncology. 2018;**16**:217

Chapter 5

Management of Blunt Cerebrovascular Injury: A Literature Review

Trung Kien Duong

Abstract

Blunt cerebrovascular injury (BCVI) is one of the most common clinical manifestations in patients with skull base trauma and severe traumatic brain injury. It is also the cause of later stroke, including ischemia and hemorrhage. Screening high-risk patients by several grading scales will support the identification and management of the complications of BCVI. Computerized tomographic angiography (CTA) and digital subtraction angiography (DSA) play a crucial role in identifying the lesion of cerebrovascular injuries. Antithrombotic therapy is the essential treatment for minimizing the risk of BCVI-related. This chapter aims to review the updated management of BCVI.

Keywords: blunt cerebrovascular injury, antithrombotic, endovascular, Denver criteria, computerized tomographic angiography, digital subtraction angiography

1. Introduction

Blunt cerebrovascular injury includes blunt macrovascular and penetrating cerebrovascular injuries, which occur in about 1% of all traumatic brain injuries, 9% in severe traumatic brain injuries, and 1–2% in the in-hospital trauma population. Most of the lesions are found in the extracranial segment of carotid and/or vertebral arteries.

Patients with cervical spine trauma, including upper cervical spine, ligamentous injuries, and traumatic subluxation placing, have the strongest association with BCVI. However, the LeFort II or III fracture and basilar skull fracture extending carotid canal patients should be alerted to BCVI. These lesions are most commonly identified in trauma patients with high-energy injury mechanisms, for example, car accidents, falling... with flexion, extension, or rotation of the neck, or a direct blow to or laceration of the blood vessels. Blunt carotid injury generally causes contralateral hemiparesis or hemiplegia, aphasia, dysphasia, or Horner syndrome. Ataxia, dizziness, or visual field deficits can be resulted from blunt vertebral injury.

The imaging modality for diagnostic BCVI still focuses on CT angiography and DSA. The standard of reference is DSA, but CT angiography becomes popular and contributes many useful characteristics of BCVI. All patients with high-risk factors for BCVI should undergo DSA as the final test for BCVI.

While the application of screening protocols is accepted generously, the treatment remains a discussion. Early identification and treatment of BCVI help reduce the rate of mortality and morbidity. Antithrombotic therapy, either with anticoagulation or antiplatelet agents, has long been accepted as the first-line of BCVI patients. However, the medication choice and the duration of treatment are still controversial.

2. Epidemiology

The prevalence of BCVI as a variant depends on the different studies. A systematic review and meta-analysis from Franz et al. [1], the incidence range of BCVI was between 0.18 and 2.7% among 122.176 blunt trauma patients. This result came from 20 studies published from 2004 to 2011.

Another prospective, observational, single-center study published in 2016 showed the incidence of BCVI was 9.2% among 228 patients with severe traumatic brain injury. The three most common risk factors included motorcycle crash, fracture involving the carotid canal and cervical spine injury [2].

The study by Hundersmarck et al. [3] showed that 0.59% of BCVI patients in 12.122 blunt trauma populations. The most popular mechanism of trauma in Hundersmarck's research was a car accident (31%) followed by fail from stairs (24%). Motor vehicle collision or other modes of transportation is also the most frequent reason of BCVI (56.1%) in a total of 1.204 patients during 10-year follow-up at a level I trauma center [4]. The result of this study showed about 42% BCVI population suffered from traumatic brain injury. The highest incidence of BCVI met in patients with cervical trauma (7.3%), followed by basilar skull fracture (1.6%), polytrauma (1.5%), and whole blunt trauma group (0.59%).

A study by Wu et al. [4] collected 1204 BCVI patients (2.5%) in a group of 47.773 blunt trauma patients. CT angiography is the key imaging to confirm the vessel injuries. The incidence of BCVI-related stroke in this research was 8.5%, the median time to stroke was 2 days (with a range of 0–12 days).

Another study by Esnault et al. [2] found that BCVI accounts for 9.2% of all severe traumatic brain injury admissions. These included 71% with carotid artery injury, 24% with vertebral artery injury, and 5% with damage to both.

The injury of carotid artery and vertebral artery in the study of Harper et al. [5] were 47 and 58%, respectively. But the difference in the incidence of stroke between internal carotid (8.8)% and vertebral injuries (3.6%) was not statistically significant.

3. Mechanisms of BCVI

High-energy injury mechanisms are confirmed as the cause of BCVI by many researchers [2, 6–8]. High-speed motor vehicle collisions are the most popular cause of BCVI, but chiropractic manipulation, direct blows to the neck, and any mechanism resulting in rapid deceleration or acceleration accompanied with or without rapid head turning was reported as the cause of BCVI. Esnault et al. [2] categorized the main mechanism of BCVI: hyperextension with contralateral rotation of the head, laceration of the artery by adjacent fractures, direct blow to the neck, and direct intraoral trauma with a hard object. This categorization is similar to the opinions of

DOI: http://dx.doi.org/10.5772/intechopen.1002873

Crissey and Bernstein in 1974. These two authors introduced 4 physiologic mechanisms which include direct blow to the neck, hyperextension with contralateral rotation of the head, laceration of the artery by adjacent fractures involving the sphenoid or petrous bone, and direct intraoral trauma with a hard device. Traumatic brain injury and skull base fractures can make easily a carotid artery injury, whereas cervical spine injury is associated with vertebral artery lesions. The most common mechanism of carotid artery injury is hyperextension caused by stretching of this artery over the lateral processes of C1 to C3.

4. BCVI screening

Some guidelines are recommended for screening patients who had high risk of BCVI, including Denver criteria and/or modified Denver criteria [9], Western Trauma Association (WTA) [7] screening recommendation, and Eastern Association for the Surgery of Trauma (EAST) [10]. The summary of screening recommendations for BCVI is shown in the **Table 1**.

Research by Biffl et al. [11] identified independent risk factors for BCVI after the follow-up of 249 patients by CT angiography. These included GCS less than 6, petrous bone fracture, diffuse axonal brain injury, and Le Fort II or III fracture. The high-risk mechanism patient with one of these circumstances was associated with a 41% risk of BCVI. The result of this study also announced that a patient with a cervical spine fracture had a 39% risk of vertebral arterial injury.

Screening for BCVI was recommended as level II by EAST in case of unexplained neurologic symptoms or arterial epistaxis after the traumatic brain injury. This guideline also gives a recommendation with III level for the asymptomatic patients who suffered from traumatic brain injury with Glasgow Coma Scale less than or equal to 8, a diffuse axonal injury, petrous bone fracture, fracture at high cervical segments [10]. The advantage of applying a screening tool helps the detection of BCVI increase versus no screening protocol [12].

A new screening model created by Japanese neurosurgeons was published in 2021 [13]. A multivariate analysis indicated 13 factors that were significantly associated with BCVI. These elements were sex (male – female), high-energy impact, hypotension on admission, Glasgow Coma Scale score below 9, injury to the face, injury to the neck, injury to the spine, injury to the lower extremity, supratentorial subdural

Signs/ symptoms	Massive hemorrhage from the neck, nose, and mouth, Cervical hematomas develop. Cervical bruit in a patient below 50 years old Focal neurological deficit Appearance of the secondary stroke on CT or MRI
Risk factors for BCVI	Maxillofacial fractures from high-energy mechanism, including mandible fracture, Le Fort II or III fractures. Complex skull, basilar skull and/or occipital condyle fractures. Cervical spine fracture or subluxation, including vertebral body fracture, transverse foramen fracture, subluxation or ligamentous injury, any fracture at C1 through C3. Severe traumatic brain injury Traumatic brain injury with thoracic injuries

Table 1.
Signs, symptoms and risk factors of BCVI.

hemorrhage, skull base fracture, cervical spine fracture or subluxation, lumbar spine fracture or subluxation, soft tissue injury of the face. When the definition of BCVI was narrowed to include only carotid and vertebral artery injuries, the AUC of the model in predicting these injuries was 0.89 (95%CI, 0.87–0.91).

5. Imaging

5.1 Digital subtraction angiography (DSA)

DSA plays a key role and standard imaging modality for the diagnosis of BCVI, but it still has some limitations. This method is an invasive, cost-effective tool, has a complication rate of 1–3% which includes vascular dissection and thromboembolism, and not provide by all trauma centers as a full-time, 24/7 service. With the development of CTA, DSA is mostly performed when an intervention is planned.

According to EAST guidelines [10], DSA was given a level II recommendation in screening BCVI. The two latest systematic review and meta-analysis study of CTA versus DSA in BCVI diagnosis suggests that CTA has reasonable specificity but low sensitivity [14, 15]. The pooled sensitivity and specificity of CTA were 64% (95%CI, 53–74%) and 95% (95%CI, 87–99%), respectively when compared to DSA. This guideline showed the estimated positive likelihood ratio, a negative likelihood ratio, and a diagnostic odds ratio was 11.8 (95%, 5.6–24.9), 0.38 (95%, 0.30–0.49), and 31 (95%, 17–56), respectively [15]. To determine the accuracy of CTA versus DSA in evaluate the lesions between BCVI carotid and BCVI vertebral, the result showed the similar in sensitivity and specificity.

5.2 CT angiography

Most of the patients who had BCVI got the polytrauma presentation. The BCVI candidates always have an indication for screening whole-body for prevention of the missing-lesions such as thoracic, abdomen, and spine. Hundersmarck et al. [3] indicated an augmentation of the dose of intravenous contrast administration flow for total body CT scanning from 3 to 6 ml/s to advance the diagnostic yield for cervical vascular lesions. Because of this remodeling, an increase in explorer incidence from 0.3 to 0.8%, from 0.9 to 2.4%, from 1.2 to 1.9%, from 4.6 to 8.5% in the whole blunt trauma group, in the polytrauma subgroup, in patients with a basilar skull fracture and in the cervical spine trauma subgroup, respectively, have been shown. These authors believe that in the setting of not scanning the total body, the patients may benefit from the modification for confirming the grade of cervical artery injuries. CTA can be used to classify and follow-up BCVIs. It can provide important decisions in the management and planning of the treatment of lesions.

In a European level 1 trauma center, the incidence of BCVI was changing between period I (using 64-slides scanner) and period II (using 256-slides scanner) [3]. During the first period, BCVI incidence was found to be 0.3% in the whole blunt trauma patients, 0.9% in the polytrauma subgroup, 1.2% in patients with basilar skull fracture, and 4.6% in the cervical spine trauma subgroup. With 256-slides scanner, the result in an increase of detected was 0.8% in the whole blunt trauma group, 2,4% in the polytrauma population, 1.9% patients with basilar fractures, and 8.5% cervical spine trauma subgroup.

CTA is a useful modality for the purpose of follow-up the BCVI patients. Wu et al. [4] suggest that CTA has the highest diagnostic yield in identifying the changing of lesions within the first 30 days after the trauma. These authors also confirm the best effect on the treatment of BCVI when CTA was performed within 30 days of injury. However, CTA has intermediate effects between 30 and 90 days, and no transformation when performed beyond 90 days, particularly in high-grade injuries.

However, the difference of channel CTA can affect the result. One- to four-slice multidetector CT angiography is neither sensitive nor specific enough for screening BCVI, and a minimum 16-channel CT angiography is available sensitive technology for diagnosis BCVI [6, 8, 10]. Kik et al. [15] showed the sensitivity and specificity that were reported at 70.3% (95%CI, 41.3–88.9) and 96.1% (95%CI, 86.5–98.9) in over 16-slice group, respectively, and 63.1% (95%CI, 46.3–77.2) 94.6% (95%CI, 61.0–99.5) in below 16-slice-CTA group, respectively. The systematic review and meta-analysis from Kik et al. only concluded that the moderate to good specificity but low sensitivity of CTA in comparison with DSA in diagnosing BCVI. Using CTA with higher channels (16–64) can not be more effective than lower channels (< 16).

The classification of BCVI in CTA or DSA was requested by Biffl et al. in 1999. It was applied for prognostication and comparison with repeated imaging (**Table 2** and **Figure 1**) [8].

A retrospective cohort study from Ares et al. [16] with 312 patients includes that DSA is more accurate and sensitive than CTA in diagnosis BCVI. The DSA helps to avoid overtreatment in up to 41% of cases (CTA false positives), and can avoid missing injuries in up to 28% of cases (CTA false negatives). They introduced a protocol with DSA after the initial trauma and repeat within 2 weeks of injury to confirm the management of BCVI patients.

Abu et al. [17] listed several lesions that can mask or mimic focal vascular injuries on CTA. It resulted from artifact to preexisting pathologies and underlying normal anatomical variants.

Artifact: such as motion, swallowing, and pulsation during the performance. Dental implant artifacts should be removed before scanning the patient.

Preexisting nontraumatic pathology: Atherosclerotic plaque that makes the vessels narrow can mimic the appearance of a vascular injury. Atherosclerotic plaque can be distinguished from intramural hematoma. We can differentiate the two lesions by MRI. Underlying vasculitis or vascular dysplasia also makes a false diagnosis.

Underlying normal anatomical variants: Segments of vessel tortuosity, redundancy, and coiling can make a mistake as a small pseudoaneurysms. Preexisting vascular duplication and fenestration sometimes can result an emulating a double-lumen sign.

Biffl et al. injury grade	Definition
Grade I	Luminal irregularity or dissection with <25% luminal narrowing
Grade II	Dissection or intramural hematoma with ≥25% luminal narrowing
Grade III	Pseudoaneurysm
Grade IV	Occlusion
Grade V	Transaction with free extravasation

Table 2.
Denver grading scale for blunt cerebrovascular injury.

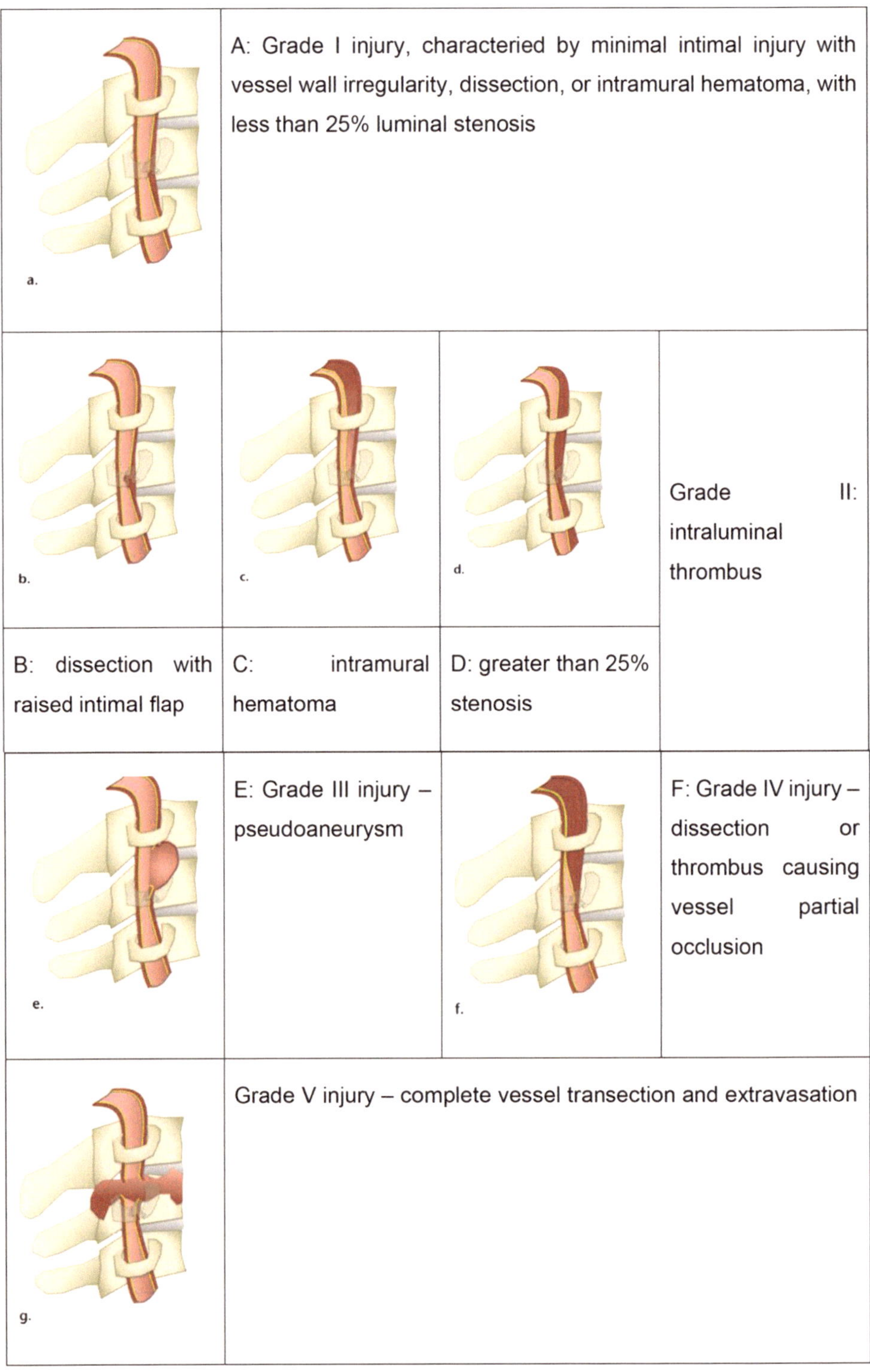

Figure 1.
Illustration of BCVI grading scale.

6. Treatment

To date, guidelines from the Western Trauma Associations [7] and EAST [10] recommend antithrombotic therapy, endovascular therapy, or surgical treatment based on the location and grade of injuries.

Recommendation from Brommeland et al. (2018) [8] suggests that a low-molecular weight heparin in antithrombotic doses within 24-48 h of the diagnosis followed by oral aspirin 75 mg daily. They also made a strong recommendation for the timing of antithrombotic therapy. Early usage as soon as possible is recommended even in the setting of severe traumatic brain injury or other solid organ injury.

In 2011, the ASA/ACCF/AHA/AANN/AANS/ACR/ASNR/CNS/SAIP/SCAI/SIR/SNIS/SVM/SVS guideline found level B for the treatment of stroke or transient ischemic attack patients with any anticoagulant agents (low-molecular-weight heparin, heparin, or warfarin) or an antiplatelet one (aspirin with or without extended-release dipyridamole, or clopidogrel exclusively) [18]. The duration of treatment lasted from 3 to 6 months after the trauma.

The practice management guideline from the Eastern Association for the Surgery of Trauma (2020) [12] suggested the benefit from the usage of antithrombotic versus no antithrombotic can decrease the risk of stroke (OR = 0.20–95%CI, 0.06–0.65 – $p < 0.0001$) and mortality (OR = 0.17–95%CI, 0.08–0.34 – $p < 0.0001$). And the guideline can not show any significant difference in the risk of stroke among patients with grade II or III injuries who underwent stenting as an adjunct to antithrombotic versus antithrombotic alone (OR = 1.63–95%CI, 0.2–12.14 – $p = 0.63$).

But the Western Trauma Association can not indicate any antithrombotic drugs for initial management. Aspirin may be available, but dual antiplatelet therapy (aspirin combined with clopidogrel) can be a safety and efficacy in a number of clinical situations [7].

Catapano et al. [19] indicated aspirin as the first-line therapy for patients with BCVI, if there were no contraindications, such as gastrointestinal bleeding, large ICH, or progression of ICH. After the treatment with aspirin, only 1/56 patients got stroke, 2/56 patients had progression of an intracerebral hemorrhage (neither required decompression) and 2/56 patients suffered from severe gastrointestinal bleeding. The result of follow-up of this aspirin group by vascular imaging showed the stable or improved levels of BCVI in 94% of patients. There were no delayed strokes or death. These authors concluded the aspirin-based management strategy for BCVI was efficacious and relatively safe.

Esnault et al. [2] made a decision to anticoagulation therapy on day 1.5, and 41% patients were indicated on arrival in the ICU. These authors believed that the latent period between injury and ischemia was observed mostly with 10–72 hours, the effect of this therapy can be easily monitored by partial thromboplastin time or anti-factors Xa activity, and in the setting of hemorrhagic complication or emergency surgery, this therapy can be quickly counteracted by protamine sulfate.

The choice of antiplatelet therapy or anticoagulation depends on the grade of BCVI, concomitant injuries, neurological symptoms, and the volume of infarcted territory at risk for hemorrhagic transformation (**Table 3**).

A study in 435 patients was treated with anticoagulation and 290 patients were treated with antiplatelet agents, Hanna et al. [20] resulted the hospital readmission rate (5.72 vs. 1.8%; $p = 0.03$), 6 months mortality rate (4.9 vs. 1.3%; $p = 0.03$) was significantly higher than in patients treated with antiplatelet agents when compared with those treated with anticoagulants. The similar result was manifested in the

Injury grade	**I**	**II**	**III**	**IV**	**V**
Dever grading system	Irregularity of vessel wall dissection or IMH with <25% narrowing	Intraluminal thrombus, dissection, small AVF, or IMH with >25% narrowing	Pseudoaneurysm	Occlusion	Transection
CTA findings	Nonstenotic luminal irregularity, intimal flap, or wall thickening with <25% stenosis	Luminal hypodensity, intimal flap, or wall thickening with >25% stenosis	Eccentric contrast-filled outpouching limited by periarterial tissue	Lack of any intraluminal enhancement, carotid occlusions (abrupt or tapered), vertebral occlusion (usually abrupt)	Irregular extravascular collection of contrast, not limited by periarterial tissues, increases in density on delayed images if obtained
Stroke incidence (%)	8% cartotid 6% vertebral	14% carotid 38% vertebral	26% carotid 27% vertebral	50% carotid 28% vertebral	100% carotid 100% vertebral
Initial therapy	Antithrombotic	Antithrombotic	Antithrombotic	Antithrombotic	Direct pressure on actively bleeding area until surgical intervention
Surgical/endovascular therapy	Not needed	Rare needed, but consider if neurologic symptoms, progression of dissection, or if refractory to therapy	Consider if symptomatic or if >1 cm	Stenting typically not beneficial, but thrombectomy ± stenting may be considered if stroke recognized within 6 h	Emergent intervention
Timing of follow-up imaging	7–10 days, then every 3–6 months until heal	7–10 days, then every 3–6 months until heal or definitive management	7–10 days, then every 3–6 months or based on symptoms	Based on symptoms	Based on symptoms
Long-term therapy	Antiplatelet therapy until healed	Antiplatelet therapy until healed or definitive surgical treatment	Antiplatelet therapy until healed or definitive surgical treatment	Lifelong antiplatelet	No data available, consider if symptomatic

AVF: arteriovenous fistula – IMH: intramural hematoma.

Table 3.
Summarize the management of BCVI based on CTA findings.

Cervical Artery Dissection in Stroke Study (CADISS) trial, however the difference did not mark a statistical significance [21].

The benefits of endovascular for patients with BCVI remain controversial because of its complication, stent predominance, and the rate of stroke. The indication of endovascular therapy includes: patients with a contraindication to antithrombotic agents, lesions that worsen or become symptomatic despite antithrombotic therapy, and lesions not amenable to surgical therapy. The grade II and III injuries should be treated by endovascular to decrease the risk of embolism and rupture by developing flow into the pseudoaneurysm. Endovascular can be performed for the grade V patients that are not surgically accessible. Patients with vessel occlusion also is the candidate of endovascular therapy to keep away from recanalization and embolic.

A conclusion from a study of Burlew et al. [22] showed that the stroke rate in the stent group (8.7%) and no-stent group (0.06%) was significantly different ($p = 0.04$). The authors suggest that intravascular stents should be reserved for the rare patient with symptomatology or a markedly enlarging pseudoaneurysm.

Surgical therapy has a limitation in the treatment of BCVI. No data, to date, can confirm the advantages of surgical performance. Carotid ligation, revascularization with direct, patch repair or bypass of the injured segment was recommended. In particular, the perioperative risk of hemorrhage may make surgical the preferred over endovascular stent, which requires antiplatelet treatment. We introduce some algorithms in management of BCVI (**Figures 2** and **3**).

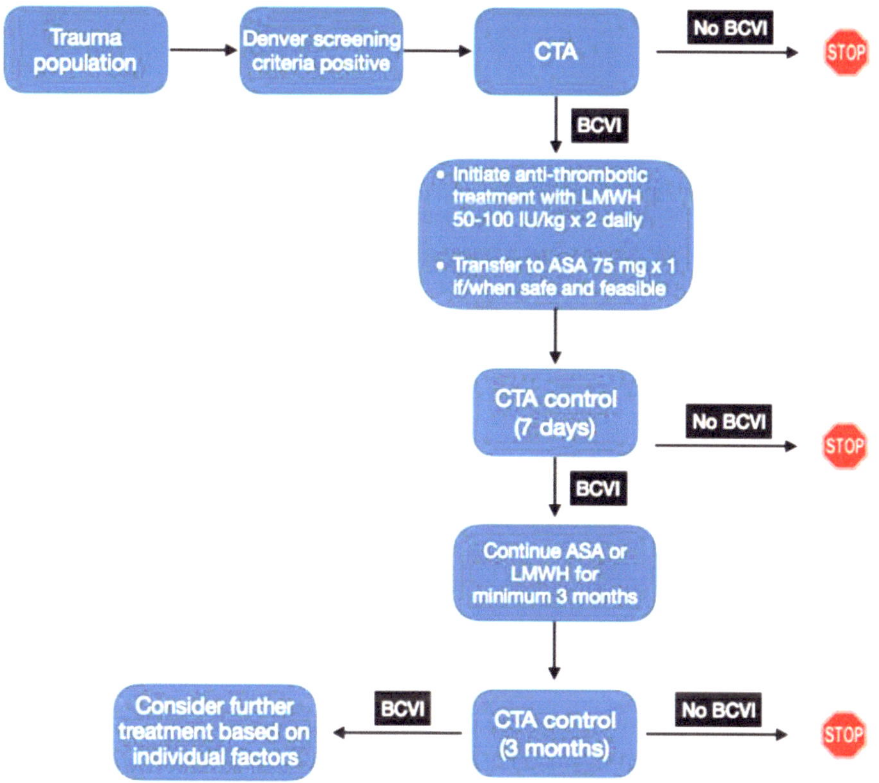

Figure 2.
A flow-diagram summarizing for management of BCVI [8].

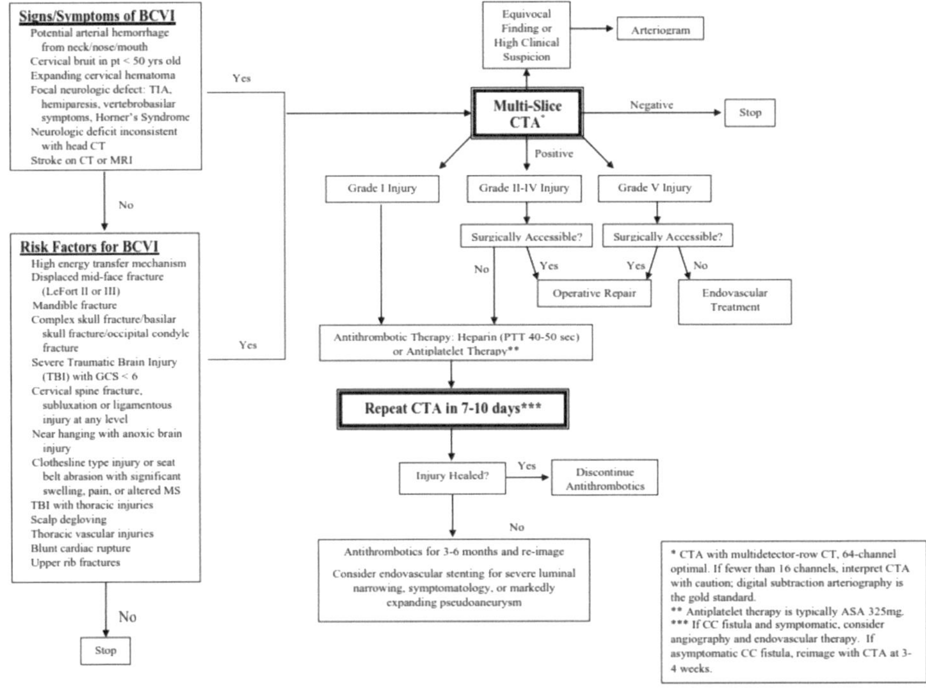

Figure 3.
The Denver health medical Center BCVI screening guideline [9].

7. Conclusion

BCVI is preventable cerebrovascular disorder by the application of screening recommendations, imaging modalities, and choosing a suitable repair therapy. CTA or DSA can be helpful to detect the morphology and location of the injuries. Early treatment of antithrombotic has been suggested to be both effective and safe, particularly in patient with minor and moderate injuries. The role of endovascular and surgical therapy remains controversial due to the lack of data.

Author details

Trung Kien Duong
Department of Neurosurgery, Hanoi, Vietnam

*Address all correspondence to: duongtkien@gmail.com

References

[1] Franz RW, Willette PA, Wood MJ, et al. A systematic review and meta-analysis of diagnostic screening criteria for blunt cerebrovascular injuries. Journal of the American College of Surgeons. 2012;**214**(3):313-327

[2] Esnault P, Cardinale M, Boret H, et al. Blunt cerebrovascular injuries in severe traumatic brain injury: Incidence, risk factors, and evolution. Journal of Neurosurgery. 2017;**127**(1):16-22

[3] Hundersmarck D, Slooff WM, Homans JF, et al. Blunt cerebrovascular injury: Incidence and long-term follow-up. European Journal of Trauma and Emergency Surgery. 2021;**47**(1):161-170

[4] Wu L, Christensen D, Call L, et al. Natural history of blunt cerebrovascular injury: Experience over a 10-year period at a level I trauma Center. Radiology. 2020;**297**(2):428-435

[5] Harper PR, Jacobson LE, Sheff Z, et al. Routine CTA screening identifies blunt cerebrovascular injuries missed by clinical risk factors. Trauma Surgery & Acute Care Open. 2022;**7**(1):e000924

[6] Rutman AM, Vranic JE, Mossa-Basha M. Imaging and Management of Blunt Cerebrovascular Injury. Radiographics. 2018;**38**(2):542-563

[7] Biffl WL, Cothren CC, Moore EE, et al. Western trauma association critical decisions in trauma: Screening for and treatment of blunt cerebrovascular injuries. The Journal of Trauma. 2009;**67**(6):1150-1153

[8] Brommeland T, Helseth E, Aarhus M, et al. Best practice guidelines for blunt cerebrovascular injury (BCVI). Scandinavian Journal of Trauma, Resuscitation and Emergency Medicine. 2018;**26**(1):90

[9] Geddes AE, Burlew CC, Wagenaar AE, et al. Expanded screening criteria for blunt cerebrovascular injury: A bigger impact than anticipated. American Journal of Surgery. 2016;**212**(6):1167-1174

[10] Bromberg WJ, Collier BC, Diebel LN, et al. Blunt cerebrovascular injury practice management guidelines: The eastern Association for the Surgery of trauma. The Journal of Trauma. 2010;**68**(2):471-477

[11] Biffl WL, Moore EE, Offner PJ, et al. Optimizing screening for blunt cerebrovascular injuries. American Journal of Surgery. 1999;**178**(6):517-522

[12] Kim DY, Biffl W, Bokhari F, et al. Evaluation and management of blunt cerebrovascular injury: A practice management guideline from the eastern Association for the Surgery of trauma. Journal of Trauma and Acute Care Surgery. 2020;**88**(6):875-887

[13] Shibahashi K, Hoda H, Ishida T, et al. Derivation and validation of a quantitative screening model for blunt cerebrovascular injury. Journal of Neurosurgery. 2021;**135**(4):1129-1138

[14] Roberts DJ, Chaubey VP, Zygun DA, et al. Diagnostic accuracy of computed tomographic angiography for blunt cerebrovascular injury detection in trauma patients: A systematic review and meta-analysis. Annals of Surgery. 2013;**257**(4):621-632

[15] Kik CC, Slooff WM, Moayeri N, et al. Diagnostic accuracy of computed

tomography angiography (CTA) for diagnosing blunt cerebrovascular injury in trauma patients: A systematic review and meta-analysis. European Radiology. 2022;**32**(4):2727-2738

[16] Ares WJ, Jankowitz BT, Tonetti DA, et al. A comparison of digital subtraction angiography and computed tomography angiography for the diagnosis of penetrating cerebrovascular injury. Neurosurgical Focus. 2019;**47**(5):E16

[17] Abu Mughli R, Wu T, Li J, et al. An update in imaging of blunt vascular neck injury. Canadian Association of Radiologists Journal. 2020;**71**(3):281-292

[18] Brott TG, Halperin JL, Abbara S, et al. ASA/ACCF/AHA/AANN/AANS/ACR/ASNR/CNS/SAIP/SCAI/SIR/SNIS/SVM/SVS guideline on the management of patients with extracranial carotid and vertebral artery disease: Executive summary. A report of the American College of Cardiology Foundation/American Heart Association task force on practice guidelines, and the American Stroke Association, American Association of Neuroscience Nurses, American Association of Neurological Surgeons, American College of Radiology, American Society of Neuroradiology, Congress of Neurological Surgeons, Society of Atherosclerosis Imaging and Prevention, Society for Cardiovascular Angiography and Interventions, Society of Interventional Radiology, society of NeuroInterventional surgery, Society for Vascular Medicine, and Society for Vascular Surgery. Circulation. 2011;**124**(4):489-532

[19] Catapano JS, Israr S, Whiting AC, et al. Management of Extracranial Blunt Cerebrovascular Injuries: Experience with an aspirin-based approach. World Neurosurgery. 2020;**133**:e385-e390

[20] Hanna K, Douglas M, Asmar S, et al. Treatment of blunt cerebrovascular injuries: Anticoagulants or antiplatelet agents? Journal of Trauma and Acute Care Surgery. 2020;**89**(1):74-79

[21] Cadiss trial investigators, Markus HS, Hayter E, et al. Antiplatelet treatment compared with anticoagulation treatment for cervical artery dissection (CADISS): A randomised trial. Lancet Neurology. 2015;**14**(4):361-367

[22] Burlew CC, Biffl WL, Moore EE, et al. Endovascular stenting is rarely necessary for the management of blunt cerebrovascular injuries. Journal of the American College of Surgeons. 2014;**218**(5):1012-1017